# OVERCOMING FEAR AND GRIEF

## My Journey of Reflection and Understanding

Sheila Malik

ISBN-978-1-7773969-0-9
ISBN-978-1-7773969-1-6

Cover design and illustrations by: Nabeela Malik

Printed in the United States of America

*My father, Mian Muzaffar Ahmad, taught me that anything is possible.*

*My husband, Mahmood, encouraged me to write and managed the publishing process.*

*My talented children, Adeela, Nabeela, Aneeqa and Saad continue to amaze me and were my inspiration and motivation to write.*

# CONTENTS

Title Page   1

Copyright   2

Dedication   3

Publishers Note   7

Understanding 6 steps to Overcome Fear and Grief   25

Step 1: Spiritual Health   26

Step 2: Physical Strength and Health   34

Step 3: Social and Emotional Health.   44

Step 4: Banking Memories   53

Step 5: Emotional Habits   56

Step 6: Reflect and Self-Reform   61

My Prayer For You   64

The Greater Jihad   65

Reflecting on How to Manage Fear and Grief   66

The Ability to Reflect and Self-Reform   67

Managing fears   74

Managing Grief   82

Planning the 6 steps   91

Journal   92

# PUBLISHERS NOTE

Allah is the Arabic name for God.

All references to the Holy Quran are written as CH(Chapter) number and Verse number. The verse numbers follow a system whereby the first verse of a chapter is "Bismillahe Ar Rehman Ar Rahim"

All prophets of Allah are written with the prayer (peace be upon him)

*O children of Adam!*
*if Messengers come to you from among*
*yourselves, rehearsing My Signs unto you,*
*then whoso shall fear God*
*and do good deeds,*
*on them shall come no fear nor shall they grieve.*
CH 7 verse 36

# Introduction

We all face fear and grief at challenging times in our lives. When we are challenged, we need to reconsider our attitudes, values, depth of faith and so many other character traits. At times, we are so heavily challenged that it may feel as though we know nothing and have no strength to discover a solution to our problems. This is when our faith is challenged the most. Since I was eight years old, I remember reflecting on why Allah allows people; and I felt they were "good" people; to suffer so much. I have always believed that everyone is "good" and that society tempts them to be "bad". However, I always saw that the people who break the rules seem to win. That is quite annoying to anyone. Even the people who break rules, get upset when others do the same. It is so confusing. What I want you to consider is; do they get away with it or do you let them get away with?

My dear reader, I want you to believe that you can solve your own problems naturally if you have faith in yourself. I want you to believe that you were born for a purpose, because you were. You have decided to read this book because you have distanced yourself from the arrogance of blame and want to solve problems rather than walk away from them. As a believer in Allah, I believe that if He decreed, I would not wake up in the morning. If I woke up, that means I have a purpose. I believe that Allah has a bigger plan which we cannot try to comprehend. That plan includes all of His creation. That plan requires His believers to be steadfast and to persevere on the righteous path. He requires us to believe in Him and to generate that faith at times of challenge and ask Him for help. Allah is the Arabic name for the Creator. There are many names for Him. In Islam, there are 100 names for Him! He is One. He has a plan. He creates and destroys as He pleases. That is the basis of our belief, right? But when we are in pain, in fear, in loss, desperate, where is He? Why do we get so confused and lost? Why do we have to turn to counseling, medication, and sometimes hospitalization? This is when we *suffer* from fear and grief.

In this book, I will share some personal experiences of myself and family and friends who are all Muslims and I will share how we found relief in Islam. I cannot claim that I have found all the answers, but I believe that I know where to find them. This belief stems from one very important day in my life. I was an inquisitive thirteen-year-old. Finally, I had a pair of glasses to correct my short-sightedness. However, there was another problem. I still struggled to read. At school, I read the front pages and the end pages and guessed the rest. I later learned that I was dyslexic, but was never assessed. My parents struggled to teach me how to read the Arabic in the Holy Quran. When I was thirteen, my father decided that they needed to try a different approach. I had so many questions about life that my mother said I would find the answers to in the Holy Quran. By-passing the Arabic, my mother gave me a Holy Quran which had the English translation beside the Arabic text and commentary and a huge index system. I loved this Quran! It was my best friend. One answer led to another question and then another answer. It was the most beautiful experience. I am a teacher and my role as such is a facilitator. I have found that Allah is the Greatest teacher since He is the Most Perfect facilitator. He facilitated my learning. I am now able to read Arabic and have read the Holy Quran many times.

My book is a practical application of what I have learned from religious teachings and from life. This book is the result of the practical guidance which I have witnessed and personally experienced through my spiritual journey of life. At half a century, I have realised that it is time I share my findings. I have also realised that my personal striving to better my life has only just really begun.

You may have read the blurb and expected that I am a serious person who has been drowning in depression and now I can tell you my story. Yes, I have faced many challenges, but, no, it did not hinder me from growing. Instead, it prepared me to a state in which I have a greater desire to learn more. At times I slowed down my learning. There were times when I regressed. Each time, it was my faith in myself and my purpose to please Allah which reignited my desire to fight on. I remember watching the original *Star Wars* movie as a child. When Obi-Wan Kenobi told Darth Vader

*"If you strike me down, I will become more powerful than you can possibly imagine."*

At the time, I was in middle school in London, England, and embarking on the life-long battle against ignorance and racism towards Muslim women. I did not wear hijab yet, but I was ethnic Pakistani and that was enough. I was also petite, needed a brace for my teeth, could barely read and had a quirky obsession with copying everything my brother did. Deep in my heart, I believed that I had special powers like Mother Theresa and one day, I would change the world.

There are many who say that womankind is a pillar of strength in every family and community, no matter how that family is composed. Each woman or girl has a significant role and her attitude supports and influences the mood and success of the family. However, in most communities, men are considered the guardian and the veto decision maker. Do men and boys have moods too? Of course, they do. Humans are male and female and they need each other and lean on each other for many things; not just having offspring. Moods are affected by our health which is affected by our hormones and chemical balance, which is regulated by our liver, which is adversely affected by our spirit and what we consume from our mouth, ears and eyes. In all my challenges, mood has played a hidden but powerful role which I wish I had addressed.

By this book, I want to show you how I was guided to a solution for a very common set of problems and conditions influenced by fear and grief. Personally, I will share experiences which enabled me to realise my true purpose in life as I grew spiritually, in my role in my many worlds as a daughter, sister, wife, mother, mother-in-law, teacher, mentor and all the other opportunities gifted to me by my Creator. For all my experiences and challenges, I am truly grateful to Allah, Lord of all the Worlds.

I will be referring to experiences of friends and relatives and students in the book also, for aspects of fear and grief which I have not experienced but have witnessed and coached them through. I trust that reading this book will launch my readers into their own quest to understand what they have gained from their life experiences and how it has been part of their life struggle. In Islam, this struggle is called the greater *jihad*.

Throughout this book, I will be referring to the Holy Quran (CH-chapter and Verse) which is the book which evolves for me as I read it throughout the course of my life. I believe that life is a journey of learning whereby each challenge is a problem-solving activity which teaches us a new lesson, enabling us to grow. My text book is the Holy Quran, since it is by name asserting that it must be read daily throughout my life. In Arabic, Qur'an means often read. Allah (Arabic. The One and Only God) created each of us. He has the design blueprint. If He has the Blueprint then He has the answers to where I should turn for help. I turn to the Holy Qur'an. I read every morning after I pray. I read one lesson which is called a *Rukku*. As I read, I consider that this is what I need to learn about today and concentrate on making a connection. The connection is always there. This is the magnificence of the Word of Allah. If you are not a Muslim but read other scriptures, I believe that you will be able to relate to Quranic guidance since we are all humans Created by Him. He loves us all. As a Muslim, I believe that Confucius, Buddha, Krishna, Jesus, Moses and all the Abrahamic prophets (Peace be upon them all) were our guides as well as many thousands of other teachers. All the messengers were guided by teachings from God. Since my religion is Islam, I will refer to the book and teachings which guide me.

*Surely, those who have believed, and the Jews, and the Sabians,[1] and the Christians — whoso believes in Allah and the Last Day and does good deeds, on them shall come no fear, nor shall they grieve.* CH5 verse70

So, my dear reader, this book is intended to walk you through a process of changing a negative mindset to a positive growth mindset; naturally. I will discuss what fear and grief are and how they are related; the consequences of fear and grief, what we should do to control these emotions, the Islamic solution, and how possible it is for anyone to apply the Islamic solution whether or not they adhere to the Islamic faith.

In the second part of this book, there is a journal workbook which can launch the journaling of your quest for a positive mindset to solve your problems. No living being is without problems. Life is full of new opportunities to learn and grow. Up to recently, I was struggling with trying to reach standards set by society. I started writing this book when I realised that I need to set my own goals and standards which I have the capacity to reach and I need to appreciate myself as a personality. I realised that I was trying too hard to please others when my only purpose is to be the best I can be. So, my dear friends, embrace your problems as a new challenge and enjoy the process of solving them. As the Prophet Luqman (The Wise One, peace be upon him), known in the west as Aesop, advised his son,

*'O my dear son! observe Prayer, and enjoin good, and forbid evil, and endure patiently whatever may befall thee. Surely this is of those matters which require firm resolve.* CH31 Verse18

May Allah help you always. Ameen.

*"And We will try you with something
of fear
and hunger,
and loss of wealth
and lives,
and fruits;*

*but give glad tidings to the patient, "*

The Holy Quran, CH2 Verse156

# What is Fear?

I am amazed to realise that it took me a very long time to understand that I must address this profound question. I had never questioned what fear is and its function and that I have fears that I was not aware of.

So, what is fear? You may have many dictionary definitions. I do not plan to be clinical here. If I reflect on this question, it echoes in my head with many, many frightening images. The more images I see, the more doors open to our worst enemy, anxiety. Fear is the root cause of stress, depression, anxiety attacks and panic. There are many psychologists and scientists who could take over at this point. They then allow the patient to talk about their biggest fears. This activity may be helpful but may also exacerbate the condition. Cognitive Behavioural Therapy is a relatively new approach which Psychologists are practicing to alleviate symptoms of depression. CBT is based on the principle that each personality needs a specialised approach based on their personal beliefs. This is the approach which Islam describes in the great *jihad* of life. As a Muslim, I would turn to the teachings of Islam in the Holy Quran. The Holy Quran is "for those of understanding who reflect."

*"Is he, then, who knows that what has been revealed to thee from thy Lord is the truth, like one who is blind? But only those gifted with understanding will reflect"* CH13 verse20

Islam requires a believer to put complete trust in Allah and His teachings. So now, the depressed and anxious patient needs to generate the brain power to show understanding, and the positive energy to reflect? That is a challenge but it is not adequate to just recite the Arabic or just read the translation. We are required to read with understanding and reflection. I realised that when my mother gave me my beautiful Quran with the translation and commentary. I have often advised friends and family who are feeling challenged to read the Holy Quran as I was advised, myself. If reading scripture is not a habit, then it is understandably challenging for someone to start reading when they are in despair. This is not as easy as it sounds. Usually, at this point, a person suffering with depression slumps back into the abyss of guilt and peeling themselves off the sofa, they attend to their mundane duties, hoping that the depression or anxiety will just disappear. It is obvious to my family when I am stressed because I start cleaning where I don't need to! But unfortunately, anxiety is waiting for me to return to the sofa. I keep my Holy Quran in the living room so that I can reach for it whenever I need to.

In the Holy Qur'an, Allah mentions fear many times through many stories of the challenges of His messengers and prophets like Jonah, Joseph and Moses (peace be upon them). Each time, He makes it clear that for believers, there is no fear and no grief. How is that possible?

*"Thereby does Allah guide those who seek His pleasure on the paths of peace, and leads them out of every kind of darkness into light by His will, and guides them to the right path." CH5 Verse17*

Fear is necessary to keep us from doing something which may cause us or others harm. If we were completely fearless then we would not restrain a child's hand reaching for a hot iron or putting a worm in its mouth. In these circumstances, fear is a valuable emotion which Allah has instilled in us which keeps us on the righteous path. Hence, fear is a guard against foolishness. We daily ask Allah to keep us safely, on the right path and save us from temptations. So, fear makes us worship, which is good. Allah places challenges on our path to test the strength of our faith and our level of obedience to Allah. Before I start a task, I remember to pray that what I do is in His name and so He guides me at those times. There are times when my negative thoughts make me feel unworthy of that guidance. At those times, looking at me on the sofa is not so hopeful.

The question is, what puts us in this state of despair? Certainly, it is when, for whatever reason, our faith is challenged. Our belief is challenged when we face a force greater than our imagination, which we fear. These days, we have so many options and mechanisms in society allowing us to change the course of our life. I am referring to social workers, counsellors, religious ministers, helplines, medical intervention and medications as well as technologies to ease our work load. With all these safety nets, why are we still afraid? Do we fear losing the things we love which make us feel secure and give us a sense of belonging? Our relationships are threatened when we lose control out of fear. So, we find it difficult to ask for help. We feel we are alone.

## Types of Fear

There are many types of fears. We react immensely at the fear caused by a traumatic event or a series of traumatic events. These events lodge themselves in our memories and are revived by triggers or repeated events. A pattern of reactions occur which create reactionary habits which can eventually become part of our personality and lead to a state of PTSD (Post Traumatic Stress Disorder). In Islam, Allah describes these habits as sins because they are steeped in negative energy, faithlessness and insincerity. Islam requires a believer to place their faith in Allah and face all events with courage. Cowardice is frowned upon in Islam.

*Those who believe, and whose hearts find comfort in the remembrance of Allah. Aye! it is in the remembrance of Allah that hearts can find comfort. CH13 Verse 29*

## Fear of People

We all remember the bullies at school. We remember how they would realise our most obvious fears and would use this to corner us into obeying them or being submissive to them. A bully is rendered useless when the victim stands up to them themselves and makes the bully look foolish. At school, children are told to tell a teacher who will then take some action to mete out consequences to the bully. However, I have found that the bully continues to be a threat to their initial victims. It is only when the victim is able to confront the bully, that the victim can forgive and move on. It is difficult for a child to face the bullies but it is possible for the child to try to empathise with the bully and forgive them. My son heard some precious advice that he should pray for a bully and tell the bully that he is praying for him. So, he did that for his bully. They are now friends! When I was at primary school in England, the principal was a very wise man. When two children had a fight or argument, they were sent to his office where they had to promise to keep a secret. My brother told me about how he was summoned because he had a fight with a boy in his class. The principal made them play a game of chess. After that he was my brother's best friend for many years. To learn how to forgive at a young age is a remarkable way learn to overcome fear.

An adult bully may be a parent, husband or wife, elder, boss, co-worker and so many other possibilities. The key here is the action of the victim. If you are that victim, you can learn to face bullies in your life by confronting them and then forgiving them. You cannot change the bully. You can only change the way you react to them. If the bully is a wife or husband then there is the added fear of rejection and guilt that you were not able to sustain a bond ordained by Allah. You are also in fear of losing custody of your children or a bond and trust with them. On reflection, it is possible to find the soul who you were in love with and forgive the behaviours and work on changing the behaviours. The key is straight talk. Be completely honest and courage will come to you. A good prayer to help you overcome the fear here is one which people rarely understand. Prophet, Muhammad (peace be upon him) said that in times of stress one should recite:

*"There is no scheme or power except with the help of Allah"*[2]

## Fear of Poverty

The fear of not having enough finances to live is a very real fear for many thousands of people across the world. Companies create incentives for high interest loans, payment plans, special credit agreements and other such schemes which encourage you to buy now and pay later. My husband has always insisted that for all purchases apart from our home, we should only buy what we have the funds available to pay for. He strongly opposed any kind of avoidable debt. This is the Islamic method of financing. However, if a Muslim does require a necessary loan from a Muslim, the lender is strictly forbidden to take any interest for the loan.

*Allah will abolish interest and will cause charity to increase. And Allah loves not anyone who is a confirmed disbeliever and an arch-sinner.* CH2 verse277

As a Muslim, I believe that Allah is Lord and provides everything, including our financial wealth. If you can make that your belief and work hard to earn money by your own labour, then your spending will be careful and budgeted.

*Those who spend their wealth by night and day, secretly and openly, have their reward with their Lord; on them shall come no fear, nor shall they grieve.* CH2 Verse 275

Sometimes it is hard to find a job in your field. I believe that whenever that has happened to me, it is because Allah wants me to learn other skills. I know many people who find it difficult to take a new career. However, I also know of many taxi drivers in Toronto who are actually highly qualified Engineers and even Doctors. I guess they have faith that better times are ahead. As a taxi driver, you can learn a lot about human suffering as your passengers reveal their thoughts in conversation.

A Muslim is also expected to pay charity, as I will discuss later. The rate for charity is a percentage of their savings, and so it takes into consideration the income of even the poorest believer. The Islamic financial system provides for everyone, so no Muslim can be in a state of poverty if they attach themselves to an Islamic community.

## Fear of Ill Health

As a child we rely on our carer to provide good nutrition and ensure good health. As adults, we are exposed to the world and are responsible for our own health. Not being medical experts, we are prone to make mistakes which can have adverse effects on our health. The media fire frightening names at us. Cancer,

Diabetes, Heart disease and Stroke, Disability, SARS, COVID-19. The list is huge. Some names are so complex that the lay-person struggles to understand what it is. The media tells us to not eat fats. Eat saturated fats. Eat Omega-3 Fish oils. Do not eat animal fats. It is so confusing! All medications have side-effects and so we are fearful of the side-effects but we need the medication. I will share what my family did to overcome this fear by focussing on nutrition and physical health and strength.

## Fear of Death

The world is immersed in a fog of the fear of death by COVID-19. This pandemic has gripped the world in a way I never imagined when I started writing this book. I had forgotten the fear of death. As I reflected on this fear which has been evident on all the news reports, I realised that some event in my past must have changed my thinking so profoundly that I have never felt that fear again. I remembered that my fear of death was strong as a child when I suffered from Asthma. I remembered gasping for air and struggling to breathe out. I remembered the anxiety attacks when I could not breathe and my dependence on my inhaler. News reports showing patients gasping for breath reminded me of that anxiety. Then I remembered the day, in my twenties, when I replaced my inhalers with homeopathic medicine and never used an inhaler again until very recently when I had bronchitis and then again, I discarded it because It did not help me. The homeopathic cure made me realise two things. Firstly, that there is a cure for every disease and secondly, that Allah opens doors of life when He decrees it. That is when I understood that I should show gratitude if I wake up in the morning by planning a busy day of creativity and generosity.

When a Muslim approaches death, it is a common practice in Islamic culture to read chapter 36 of the Holy Quran called *Yasin.* Although we read the Holy Quran every day all our lives, it intrigues me why this chapter is read to such a helpless being. Yasin means the perfect human being. It refers to the Holy Prophet of Islam, Muhammad (peace be upon him). He was sent to teach us how to live a fulfilling life. All prophets were sent to teach us how to live. The chapter reminds believers that our life and death is in Allah's hands and that there is a life after death and other events which we have been prepared for. If we have believed in Him and follow the teachings of our religion intelligently, and live every day in His service, then we are prepared for death and the events after that. Our future is eternal after death and Allah will be pleased with us and will forgive what we beg for forgiveness for. This is how we can overcome a fear of death.

*It was said to him, 'Enter Paradise.' He said, 'O, would that my people knew,*

*'How graciously my Lord has granted me forgiveness and has made me of the honoured ones!'*
CH36 verse 27-28

## Fear of Allah

This book is focussed on a fundamental belief in Allah or God the Creator. *Fear God* is a very familiar phrase for believers of any faith. I love Allah. I also fear Allah. So how does that work? It is similar to how I fear my family members. I do not want to upset them or fail to do what they need from me. Allah wants us to find and stay on the right path. But what if I sin. That is such an old-fashioned word now. A sin is any action which displeases Allah or hurts any of Allah's creation in any way. So, fear in Allah is fear of displeasing Him by hurting any of His creation in any way. This is the only fear which is useful and must stay in our hearts.

I remember at Primary School assemblies, singing a song called *"O Sinner Man"* There are many versions of the song. I remember learning about sin from this song. In the song, the sinner man is asked;

*"O Sinner Man,*
*Where you gonna run to,*
*All on that Day"*

I realised that I cannot escape sin. I may hide something from my family members. I can even sometimes hide some things from my mother. Although she has a very strong connection with Allah and so she knows what I am experiencing by dreams and then she calls me and, of course she knows the truth. However, according to the song, my eight-year old heart learned that you cannot hide from God. I remember imagining the tress swaying in my local park and how they whispered to the world that I had lied about my brother to avoid getting into trouble.

*"Run to the trees,*
*The trees are a swaying,*
*All on that Day"*

That Day is referring to the Day of Judgement when all mankind will be assessed and sent to relevant levels of Heaven or Hell. This belief is essential for justice. Allah is just. I learned at this young age that the best way to avoid hell was to be loving to all and to hide any negative feelings. My fear remained a fear that anyone may find out what secrets I am hiding about the sins I commit. When

I learned the vital prayer for seeking forgiveness from Allah, I felt liberated because I was, and now am able to determine my intentions and fix the problem before it escalates. Sometimes these sins can be very subtle mistakes. If I have hurt someone, it is a sin. There are no big sins or little sins. They are all sins. There are no sins which I can blame others for. If I did a sin, that was my action and I am responsible for it. To repent, I must acknowledge that my action was a sin and then I must intend to not repeat it. Then I can pray:

*"I beg pardon from Allah for all my sins and turn to Him"*

How can I avoid sin? Before I embark on a challenging event, I pray:

*"I seek refuge in Allah from Satan the accursed, In the name of Allah, the Gracious, the Merciful"*

By this prayer, I acknowledge that I need Allah all the time and I am helpless without Him. Satan is the name of the evil being who challenged Allah that he would mess with humankind and tempt them all to sin. By acknowledging this temptation to sin and asking Allah for forgiveness, we can overcome this fear of Allah.

**Many Fears**

There are many other fears which you will be familiar with. The key is to reflect on how you face the fear and how you gain strength of courage to face it. If, my dear reader, you can relate to this situation and know that fear is an issue, I hope and pray that I can provide you some hope. God-Willing. In the second part of this book, you will find activities to help you relate to your fears and overcome them. You can create your own journal to set you on the path to strength and understanding. I am not fearless. I know how to overcome each fear as I face it. My greatest fear is the fear of displeasing my Creator.

# What Is Grief?

Throughout life, we are tested with losses. The reaction to the loss is grief. Grief causes psychological stress.

## Death

This grief may be loss of life of a relative, friend or personality or an animal whom we were personally attached to. The level of personal connection determines the sensation of loss. As I grew up in England, I lived with my parents but no grandparents. As a substitute for my grandparents, we adopted our parents' uncles and aunts. When they passed away, I grieved as if they were my real grandparents, however, when I was asked how I was related, that relationship was belittled and I was told to get over it. Of course, I could not, so I grieved alone. For each "grandparent", I yearned to join the "real" family and grieve with them, but I could not justify it. When my real grandmother passed away, I felt very little grief since I hardly knew her. I was judged for being so uncaring. These feelings are from the heart. They do not need to be justified. They just need to be felt and soothed over. This is a necessary piece of understanding for carers since many people have migrated for various reasons and many people are living away from their native environments. Hence there must be many more people who have "substitute relatives". It is quite irrelevant who the person is on the family tree, if there is a loss then there will be feeling of grief which needs to be addressed in order to overcome the grief.

## Traumatic Separation

Separation may be due to war or migration. It may be an agreed separation of parents, siblings, partners and friends which can also be very grievous. Depending on how strong the connection, the separation can be a devastating loss, causing much pain from negative feelings like guilt, anger and low self-esteem. If the separation is not in your control, then it is more frustrating and grievous since you also lose the power to stop it. The loss of separation can also involve the loss of belongings and environment change. I worked with one lady who had her child after the separation, but due to custody laws, the child spent 5 years connecting with her father. Her heart must be so confused about her relationship. She will need to understand her father one day and that wound will need to be healed somehow. The mother has needed to be very compassionate and patient but has expressed that Allah has supported her throughout the process. Islam enforces rules of custody but also teaches us to be compassionate and Prophet Muhammad (peace be upon him) endorsed an amicable settlement rather than an argumentative tug of love. Allah created the child and so He wants the parents to take care of the child. Generally, in life there is a continuum of losses and gains. These are all to test our independence and resilience. We need to remember the lessons we learned and then let go and Islam reminds us to realise that we will also go one day so we need to overcome this grief by resigning to the Will of Allah.

## Disasters

Many people have suffered loss due to a disaster such as fire, theft, accidents, war, epidemics and natural disasters. There is much grief associated with such events and whole communities may be suffering PTSD (Post-Traumatic Stress Disorder) together. There may be a combination of losses; such as loss of life, property, livelihood, relationships and others. In some countries, families are divided due to religion or citizenship and ethnic origin. History has shown how compassionate people are at these times and we see this frequently with refugees in Canada. The pain is personal and to overcome it, must be addressed personally.

## Chronic Illness or Hospitalization

If you or a loved one are diagnosed with an illness or inflicted with one which requires immediate hospitalization, then there is a feeling of loss and grief. This is the loss of control of your life. The entire change of routine and diet and lifestyle can be as traumatic as loss of life. Although the illness is limited to the patient, it is now recognised that the family suffers much and may need their own therapy to cope with the life changes involved. If there is an incurable chronic illness, then the care duties can completely change the life of family members in many ways. There may be a loss in finances, social access, availability of time, access to respite and many other constraints which the patient may not be aware of. My mother-in-law was always more upset about inconveniencing us than her own pain when she was ill. For someone like that, it can feel very embarrassing for them when there is a need for paramedics or doctors out-of-hours. To overcome the grief of incapacity, we need to accept the compassion of loved ones.

## Abuse

Physical, emotional, sexual or any other type of abuse is another way in which you may lose control of your life. You are living in fear and loss. There is a loss of trust. There are many news reports of such incidents but there are many more unreported cases of such abuse in the most unexpected cases. I am referring to domestic violence, child abuse, racism, ageism, sexism, and all the other types of discrimination which society is now, humbly, beginning to address from its roots.

I introduced that I suffered racism as a child. My earliest memory of this is when I wanted to take part in a school nativity play in my primary school in London, England. I was 7 years old. My friends and I all auditioned. We were all of South Asian ethnic origin. We were offered the part as sheep with the 'Shepherds who watched the flocks at night'. We were happy. We did not realise how racist the decision was until we started rehearsals. We were all brown sheep. We had to sing "We are sheep, we haven't any brains at all" My self-esteem was crushed and we had to face this in the school yard at recess. We trusted our teachers. We were only 7 years old! How many people in the world still face more severe racist abuse?

When we consider sexual abuse, a whole spectrum of events come to mind. That abuse is relative to the level of shame in the heart of the victim. As children we learn about shame. We learn about boundaries. The medical world only recognises sexual abuse relative to the norms set by western society. For a Muslim child, his or her body is sacred and the feeling of shame is embedded in the heart at a very early age. Allah teaches us that by age 7, a child must be respected and given a separate sleeping area and must observe habits of chastity and modesty. Consider the case of a little 7-year-old girl who suffered from frequent urine infections and when hospitalised required an intrusive medical procedure. The male doctor was completely unaware of her need for a female doctor. She bore the horror of that trauma silently through her adult life, marriage, motherhood and various illnesses. She was not aware of the impact of her fears on her relationships until she recalled the childhood event and addressed it by forgiving the event as an unintentional mistake. The campaign against public sex-education rages on for the same reason. Allah tells us that such an education is necessary but within the safety of the lap of parents.

Certainly, there are cases of extreme harshness and severity all around us. There is ease after suffering. That is a promise of our Creator. It rests with the individual to find that peace through faith in Him and so, overcome the pain of grief.

# UNDERSTANDING 6 STEPS TO OVERCOME FEAR AND GRIEF

All of the types of fear and grief may be overcome by faith and inner strength. It makes us feel weak and we are taken by surprise. In our weak state our body reacts immediately with the fight or flight response. Our success depends on several factors, and steps need to be taken to balance those factors;

1. Spiritual Health
2. Physical Strength and Health
3. Social and Emotional Health
4. Banking Memories
5. Emotional Habits
6. Reflect and Self-Reform.

In my journey, I have addressed all of these factors and have learned more than I imagined possible. Life is about trials and crises and how we face them and find solutions. Islam tells us that these trials are to enable us to learn and get closer to Allah by turning to Him and pleasing Him. We can pray for sometimes many years as the prophet Job (peace be upon him) did.

*"And We will try you with something of fear and hunger, and loss of wealth and lives, and fruits;*
*but give glad tidings to the patient, "*
CH2 Verse156

So now let us look more closely at each factor and tease out exactly who we are and how we can heal. By addressing each factor, the daily Islamic routine has helped me to overcome fear and anxiety and opened new doors of hope and success according to new goals. Although I was born as a Muslim, I did not fully understand what it meant to be a Muslim until I was in my teens and my mother gave me the English translation of the Holy Quran. I hope that what I share serves to clarify how Allah is a living communicator and loves us, His creation.

# STEP 1: SPIRITUAL HEALTH

**Prayer**

In the Islamic way of life, prayer is essential. It is a habit which I have lost and gained many times. We wake for prayer and then pray at specific times of the day. This routine gives our day structure and purpose. We wake to the sound of a melodious call encouraging us to pray in order to be successful. In the morning call, we are advised in this call that *"prayer is better than sleep"*. This call is the *Adhan* which we hear in the Arabic language at every prayer time. For me it is *Adhan* recorded on my phone alarm.

We are advised to get out of bed, wash thoroughly according to a prescribed process and then go to the mosque so we can pray with others. Hence, we begin the day by meeting our friends and praying to Allah.

Muslim women are encouraged to, but are not expected to go to the mosque because we may need to attend to our dependent children or elders. However, we are required to pray at the same time and so, we can create a congregation with our dependents at home in a designated prayer area. I set my area in the living area in my open-planned main floor. This ensures that everyone is involved and unites us as a family. As the day progresses, there are five obligatory prayer times and the prayers differ slightly in length and content. As well as those, we are encouraged to recite short prayers for specific needs in our daily activities.

Allah has prescribed so many specific steps for our benefit because He loves us and cares for us and He knows what is good for us according to the blueprint which only He has full access to. However, He has also made some accommodations for any special needs or illness.; if you cannot stand, you can sit and if that is difficult, you can lie down. If we look in detail at the procedures prescribed, it is amazing how many benefits are provided in each step.

**Call to Prayer**

The call to prayer, known as *Adhan*, is performed by a *Muedhin*. He has an attractive and powerful voice and makes the melodious call loudly so that all can hear. He reminds the believers to come to pray for prosperity, to recognise the One God, and to worship Him.

As humans, we may idolise many people. Firstly, our parents or guardians are infallible until we become conscious that they do actually make mistakes. We obey and fear upsetting our parents or guardians. We do all we can to please them. We effectively learn how to worship in this stage. Then we idolise our teachers and celebrities from whom we learn and grow our personality. Eventually, they let us down in some way but we have been in fear or in awe of them for many years. The relationships steadily all experience the same fate but Allah remains the One. Five times a day, we are reminded to keep our focus on Allah and fear shirk (idolising any other being). If you think of all the fears you have, they all connect with someone who we idolise. The simple act of humanising them, could eliminate many of our fears. Humanising them could also make it plain to us that they may not have all the answers or their answers may not be timeless. That is why the *Adhan* reminds us that prayer is the key to prosperity and the true wealth is our level of belief in this.

By acting on the call, we leave our activity and proceed to the mosque or prayer area and join other worshippers. These days, *Adhan* is not always delivered so that it can be heard outside the mosque to respect non-Muslims in the area. Many Muslims have *Adhan* programmed in the cell phone or alarm clock. I find that much more effective. For stress relief, the sound of *Adhan* is powerful. Leave the stress behind for a while and it loses much of its power and our fear appears petty.

## Ablution

Before we pray, we must wash by performing *wudhu* (Ablution). The steps for *Wudhu* are described in the Holy Quran CH 5 Verse 7. There is also a prayer to be read while washing which was taught to us by Prophet Muhammad (peace be upon him)

*"Oh Lord make me of those who repent and purify themselves."*

Many of our fears are related to our health and well-being. The steps of *Wudhu* are performed at least five times a day. We wash our hands to cleanse from dirt and germs depending on what we have done with our hands. We wash our arms and feet and head and face. We rinse our nose and mouth and prevent the collection of germs travelling into our digestive system. We perform *Ghusl* whereby we wash after attending the toilet and thereby prevent any germs entering the digestive and urinary tracts and the genital area. While we wash, we also massage and cool the back of the neck, forehead and the elbows which are pressure points and this relieves stress. We wash our feet which cools them and our blood. So, the act of *Wudhu* is a means for keeping healthy and preventing fearful diseases.

## Steps of Wudhu

Each step is repeated 3 times thoroughly.

1. Wash hands,
2. Wash nostrils and mouth and face
3. Wash arms, head, ears and neck
4. Wash feet and ankles
5. Wash hands

At the time when the world was inflicted with SARS or the COVID-19 pandemic, the public was constantly being advised to wash frequently and thoroughly.

## Preparing for Prayer

Having enjoyed the beautiful experience of ablution, we are expected to prepare the prayer area. I ensure that my clothes are clean and we must be dressed modestly. I lay down a clean special prayer mat and assemble my family in straight rows. Our shoulders are touching and our feet are aligned. Contact in this spiritual state triggers the chemical, oxytocin in the brain which reduces our pain and we feel a sense of love and belonging. Touch also causes the level of cortisol, the stress hormone, to drop. Our body is grounded and ready for worship.

## Daily Prayer Routine

We recite prayers at each significant posture, guiding our thought process. The prayer can be understood when linked with the posture. When standing I declare the prayers in praise of Allah's Greatness, Mercy and Graciousness as if I am telling the world. When bowing, I make myself humble. When sitting, I praise His messengers and declare my faith in Allah and His guidance as if I am a student. I beg forgiveness for my deviance from this guidance, humbly. Finally, I prostrate in complete helplessness with my personal prayers and expressions of gratitude as if I am begging. The prayer ends with a greeting of peace to those who prayed beside me. This whole meditative process takes 5 to 15 minutes and then can be extended with extra prayers if I wish.

**Fig 1.2 Postures of Prayer.**

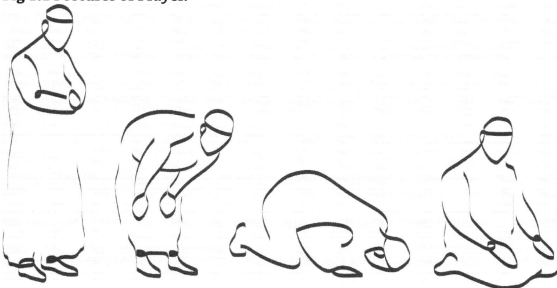

To engage in this meditation five times a day at dawn, afternoon, late afternoon, sunset and at night, should be adequate spiritual nourishment to calm and regulate my emotions and make me resilient. In the whole routine, meditation and actions combine to relax the mind, body and spirit. The words of prayer engage the mind to focus on important aspects of faith. Each prayer directs me towards a positive, growth mindset. If I desire, I can pray in this way at other times as a bonus.

As a Muslim adult, when we truly reflect on the words of prayer and the action of prayer, we realise the blessings of this form of meditation and reflection. I do not pray because Allah needs my prayers. I pray because I need to speak to Allah. I am naturally focussed on my personal needs and wellbeing. I am in awe at how the Merciful Allah has prescribed prayer as a treatment for human weaknesses. Every minute detail is a treatment for a condition which we may or may not be aware of.

Why, then, is there scope for anxiety? This is the key to all ailments. Sincerely, I cannot remember ever being engaged so purely in prayer that I have benefitted fully from it. In the state of prayer, frequently, my mind creeps away into other thoughts and I am distracted by my fears. Being human, I am easily bounced back from the spiritual realm. Simple anxieties such as "did I switch off the stove?", "what is my toddler doing in the washroom?", "I forgot to pay the gas bill" and the list can go on. So, it is a blessing that there are five opportunities to pray for my long list of needs and wants. If I am in a depressive state or I am unwell, the probability of my being distracted increases. In a depressive state, I may not even feel that I want to talk to Allah. I may feel so hopeless that I begin to doubt and drift further away. As mentioned earlier, this is when faith is challenged and fears may become more powerful than faith in Allah. This is when there is a need for others to help and notice that there is a change in mood and routines and the desire to come to the prayer area or the mosque. This is why there are extra blessings if the believing people worship in congregation together. If the depressed or anxious soul is left in solitude, the hopelessness may escalate and the consequences may be destructive.

## The Power of Prayer

During the prayer time, a believer is engaged in a dialogue with the Creator and Sustainer of life. The believer is asking for many things. I praise Allah for being everlasting, All Powerful, The Sustainer, The Provider, The Gracious, The Merciful and many other attributes of the 100 that He has taught us about Him. I ask Him to keep me good and on the right path under His guidance. I ask for all I need for my life on Earth. I ask for the good health of myself and my loved ones. I ask for forgiveness for my mistakes; known or unknown to me. I ask for His forgiveness and love for all those who have inspired me from Prophet Muhammad (peace be upon him) and all the other prophets, to my dependents and those who have made my life fruitful.

Then with all these prayers, why anxieties and fears? It is easy to believe that all your prayers will be accepted. In Islam, we attribute all power to Allah. As such, it is His will that decides Divine Decree. If Allah does not wish to grant the prayer, then it will not be granted. When my father was at the final stage in his cancer, of course, I prayed in anguish that he would gain some strength so that the doctors may use laser treatment and then he would recover. However, I was also aware that if Allah has decreed his end, then my father would not recover. For a believer, the prayer is a way of asking and begging for what he thinks is good. Similarly, a child may beg his mother to let him touch a rose, but his mother may hold him back because of the thorns he has not noticed.

In a state of fear and depression, you may ask Allah for something once or twice and anticipate that it should happen. It is frustrating when it does not happen. Sometimes, we can forget that our time-scale of years are just like milliseconds for the Creator. So, we have to be patient. You need to keep praying and begging.

This can be challenging in isolation and that is why congregational prayer is such a blessing. When you pray with a companion, they notice your mood and may even pray for you if you ask them. Sometimes a complete stranger at the mosque may be a source of guidance. For this reason, Allah manifests Himself as a Living, Sustaining God. That guiding friend may be sent as an angel to provide guidance from scripture and beliefs and rituals which will enable you to overcome your anxieties.

## Reading Scripture

In religion, believers are provided scripture to read as a source of solutions to life problems. Many scenarios are narrated which are common to all people, throughout time. Believers are encouraged to educate themselves from any source and to reflect on what is learned. For a Muslim, these scriptures are The Holy Quran, Hadith (sayings of the Prophet) and Sunnah (actions of the Holy Prophet Muhammad (peace be upon him)

### The Holy Quran

A Muslim is advised to read two lessons of the Holy Quran after the morning prayer every day. Before reading the Holy Quran, we are required to do the same ablution as for prayer, so many Muslims like to read the Holy Quran immediately after prayers. In the Holy Quran, Allah recommends to us to recite the Holy Quran after the morning, *Fajr* prayer.

A Muslim may dip into the Holy Quran at any other time in the day as much as they like. As a teenager, I enjoyed reading a translation which had a detailed index system. I was able to follow my train of thought and find many answers as the notes led me to various scenarios related to the issue I was interested in. Now, technology has made it even more accessible with remarkable websites for interactive Holy Qurans.

### Hadith and Sunnah

Believers are required to be busy in the day with hard work to earn their livelihood and contribute to society with their labour and their knowledge and charity. All these acts are considered worship in Islam. We learn about theses habits from The Sayings and Actions of the Holy Prophet Muhammad (peace be upon him). Islam is recognised as supported by five distinct pillars.

Prophet Muhammad (peace be upon him) said, *"Islam is built upon five: to worship*

*Allah and to disbelieve in what is worshiped besides him, to establish prayer, to give charity, to perform Hajj pilgrimage to the house, and to fast the month of Ramadan."*

If any of these pillars become weak or break, then the faith of the believer will be compromised. A Muslim should try to uphold each pillar, however only if there are the physical means. These pillars are;

## Five Pillars of Strength in Islam

All Islamic practices are based on the Holy Quran, Sayings of the Prophet (Hadith) and practices of the Holy Prophet (Sunnah). The Five Pillars stem from this base. They give every Muslim immense strength of faith.

**1.Creed.** This is a personal declaration of faith in Allah as the One Creator and The Prophet Muhammad (peace be upon him).

**2.Daily Prayer.** This is the ritual prayers at prescribed times, five times a day as I have described earlier.

**Fig 1.3 The Five Pillars of Islam**

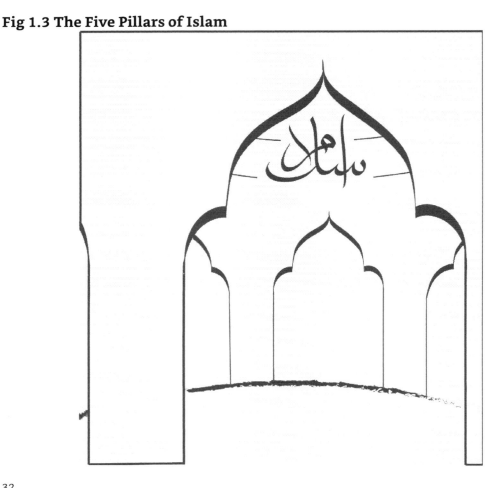

**3.Charity.** This particular charity is called *Zakaat*. *Zakaat* is required from every Muslim man or woman who has savings. It reminds us that we have been gifted with wealth so that we can learn to share and be grateful. This act makes a community strong. The power of love is strengthened by this act of charity which benefits the receiver and the giver. It is beneficial to also give other types of charity, called *sadqa*, especially at challenging times. My mother always showed me how to give *sadqa* at any time of trial in a charity box or to a poor person or as donations to specific causes to overcome any challenges.

**4.Fasting.** This is referring to the fasting in the Islamic month of *Ramadhan* for those who are physically able. For a month, physically able Muslims are required to fast by not consuming any food or drink from dawn to dusk. There are many benefits to fasting and so a Muslim may fast at other times in the year also, for the purpose of self-reform, self-control of desires and passions, many physical and spiritual and emotional benefits and, yes, it's a good weight loss strategy! Our appetite influences a desire for other things including relationships. Restricting the appetite can also regulate our appetite for belongings, events and relationships. A month or so of fasting is prescribed in all religions once a year but if the intention is to reduce the appetite for physical or mental health reasons, then fasting can be on a daily or weekly basis. If the eating times are replaced with prayer, worship, meditation or just keeping busy, then new, healthier habits can be formed.

**5.Pilgrimage.** This is the annual pilgrimage to Mecca in the Islamic month of Hajj for those who can afford it. There is a set program of events which constitute the pilgrimage. A Muslim will try to do this when he or she is physically and financially able and free of responsibilities. Any Muslim can perform the *Hajj*.

Muslims travel to Mecca at all times of the year to perform an optional, shorter pilgrimage called *Umrah*. This pilgrimage is also for the purpose of cleansing the soul but is not as powerful as Hajj. I was privileged to be able to perform Umrah twice in 2016. I went with my husband. The Umrah only took 2 hours to perform but in those two hours I witnessed many personal miracles. Perhaps I will publish my Umrah diary one day.

Our spiritual well-being is essential for the process of overcoming fear and grief. Developing the habits of worship in our daily routine enables us to face challenges with Allah watching over us. In the journaling section of this book, you will be reflecting on these aspects of your spirituality.

# STEP 2: PHYSICAL STRENGTH AND HEALTH

Our physical body is a gift from Allah which enables us to engage in actions to express our thoughts and feelings and to provide for our daily needs. The Holy Quran mentions body parts in 63 verses for various reasons. Most often mentioned are the hands and heart. As I mentioned earlier, Allah has the blueprint to our body and so He is our best doctor and He has mercifully described the importance of many parts in the Quran for our guidance. We must use all those parts in a positive manner to have the most productive and positive life on earth.

That is not to say that a person who has physical disabilities or limitations is not able to fully express themselves. A person may appear to be physically challenged, but when you interact with them, it is apparent that Allah has compensated for each inability with an alternative ability which may even be such a strength that it excels the abilities of "normal" or typical people.

Allah has provided specific guidance regarding our physical health and strength. The human body demands activity and change. The day can be a positive experience if we are active and creative within the limits of possibility. Any excess or lack of activity or creativity may lead to feelings of failure and hence grief. In the journaling section of this book, you will be reflecting on these aspects of your life.

A positive mindset may be achieved with

1. Healthy food,
2. Quality sleep,
3. Positive social interaction and
4. Exercise.

Anxiety is the result of a negative mindset, whereby experiences are viewed only regarding their damaging effects and so the creative effects of that experience may be ignored. This collection of negative experiences shapes the mind so that the mind is in a constant state of loss and is anxious to swim out of it. However, due to the negative mindset, the body is accustomed to being in a state of anxiety and is filled with fight or flight hormones which can be very damaging to health. In order to come out of this state, the conscious mind needs to decide to change its state and develop new viewpoints to create a positive mindset. This process, in Islam, is a constituent of the greater *jihad*.

If we think about the sofa scenario, we all have experienced a time when we are "stuck" to the sofa. We may even be hungry but will not want to get up and prepare or even find food. That state of depression or anxiety, deprives us of the ability to take care. We need to be taken care of. Now, if you have friends who you have a habit of meeting regularly or even just texting regularly, they will know what state you are in. They may offer to take you out. Going out is usually what the doctor prescribes and there are good reasons for that. The thought that you may have social interaction releases the chemical serotonin to the brain which is a very important anti-depressant. That boost peels you off the sofa and you start to think of what to wear, where to go, what to do, how to get there, who to be with. Once the momentum has started, progress is possible. So, how can you spend that time of physical and social activity?

1.Visit a friend
2.Visit a place of worship or community centre
3.Go shopping
4.Play a sport
5.Workout at a gym
6.Walk in the park or open space
7.Get a physically challenging job
8.Pursue a hobby.

All of these activities require some motivation to get started and then when it is routine, become the motivation to keep going. My first experience of this was post-natal depression.

Before I became a mother, I was teaching full time as the science lead in a thriving middle school. I had friends and responsibilities. I dressed smart and made healthy meals. I had a great social life and spiritually I was highly motivated and well nourished. Then, suddenly, my life was taken over by my adorable baby. Diapers, feeding, sleep deprivation and housework. I was housebound and not in any kind of control of my body. I had been in the habit of a very strict schedule and now didn't even know where my clock was. My only regulator was my husbands' routine. In this situation, my saviour was the sturdy stroller we had invested in for baby. I had appointments with doctors and health visitors for the baby and me at locations within walking distance.

I would dress smart and pack a bag and plan more than just the appointment. Baby in the stroller, I marched out on my new adventure. Perhaps if I had given more importance to the prayer times, I may not have been so lost.

There were times that I slumped into the sofa but the appointments pulled me off again. I learned from that experience that keeping a diary and scheduling events keeps you safe from any kind of depression, but I later learned that over planning can lead to anxiety because deep rooted in my mind was fear. I had conquered the depression of my grief of losing my freedom, but it was replaced with a fear of making mistakes. I was unaware that this fear was lurking deep inside my mind and had grown due to my new responsibilities as a wife and mother. With each new child, that fear mushroomed secretly inside my mind and only started to diminish when the children started school and I regained some freedom and time to schedule for myself again. I must reassure you that those early years of motherhood were the best memories of my life and I would not trade them for anything. The fear was an essential element in the growth of my positive mindset.

*And We have enjoined on man concerning his parents — his mother bears him in weakness upon weakness, and his weaning takes two years — 'Give thanks to Me and to thy parents. Unto Me is the final return.* CH31 Verse15

## Achieving a Positive Mindset

### 1.Healthy Food

**The Modern Diet**

When I talk to friends who have some kind of health issue, the first thing they say is that they need to get fit and lose weight. The problem is that they lack motivation. The brain is drained and malnourished and so there is little motivation to change old habits. We are what we eat. All our cells need a variety of nutrients to enable them to function in the intended way. The brain instructs the body to acquire that nourishment from wherever it can. In the journaling section of this book, you will be reflecting on these aspects of your diet and how you manage your pantry.

Perhaps a hundred or so years ago, there were not these problems at such a level. It certainly has escalated. It is becoming common belief that the culprit is technology. Whereas it is asserted that technology is a means to improve the quality of life, it is increasingly proving to diminish our quality of life. When we bite into an apple, we hope that the body will be nourished with lots of iron and vitamin C as well as many other nutrients. We hope in vain. The apple we bite into is probably GMO. It has been sprayed with chemical pesticides. It has been coated with wax to prevent bruising in transit.

Where I now live, there is only a short 3-month period when we can obtain local produce. For 9 months we must manage with imported food. So, is that apple a day going to keep the doctor away? Our healthcare system is overstretched with chronic diseases and annual viruses and infections. The organic business is thriving and some Canadians dream of retirement so they can become "snowbirds" and migrate for the winter to exotic locations around the world.

The internet is teeming with sites about various diets. The diet which best fit the needs of my family was a natural, seasonal, alkali diet. The acidity was obviously interfering with digestion which was causing stress and hence anxiety. To counter this, it was necessary for me to be aware of what I eat and to balance my meals so that I consume foods which cleanse my body of the toxins which I am obliged to consume. I am also obliged to take supplements to compensate for the impoverished diet of the non-productive seasons here.

If you are in a climate where the growing season is longer, I would advise that you take up the hobby of growing your own fruit and vegetables using organic seeds. The activity will keep you busy, active, alert, engaged, happy and excited. You don't need a large space. You can use pots on a patio or veranda. It is also a social activity and will lead to social events when you choose to share the food you grow. If you love your garden, then you will have a source of joy and positive emotions.

**My Family's Diet**

I only truly became aware when a member of my family was inflicted with a chronic illness. We turned to Allah's guidance.

*Now let man look at his food: How We pour down water in abundance, Then We cleave the earth — a proper cleaving —Then We cause to grow therein grain, And grapes and vegetables, And the olive and the date-palm. And walled gardens thickly planted, And fruits and herbage, Provision for you and your cattle.* CH80 verses 25-33

The first step we took was to start juicing. We started juicing with our cold press slow juicer. We started to research the nutritional value of all our food. WE DISPOSED OF OUR MICROWAVE!!! This was a great step for us. We started to prepare nutritious meals as freshly as possible. My husband built a raised garden and I started to grow many of the juicing ingredients for our cleansing, green juice. This very small garden yielded a delightful crop throughout the limited Canadian growing season. We reduced the quantity of food we cooked so that it was completely consumed at the meal and very little went into the fridge.

The next step I took was to analyse how many ingredients came out of a packet or box. We stopped buying cereals and I made it a habit to make organic oatmeal, or semolina *halva* (semolina pudding) with dates and nuts or barley pudding for breakfast as well as eggs and the great green juice. We focussed on breakfast. Our next step was to focus on the consumption of lunch. My children were always responsible for assembling lunches for school but now they were responsible for cooking the contents also. My 10-year-old son was inspired to learn to cook and now at 14 is more reliable than me for some of his recipes. They were only permitted one packaged item a day.

Our next step was for me to look at the ground spices which I used in my meals. I replaced almost all of them with whole spices and invested in a hand grinder (pestle and mortar) so that for all meals I was using freshly ground spices. The flavours were exciting and the health benefits were immediate. Our meal-times became increasingly joyful and hopeful as we became determined to become strangers to our doctors.

Our next step was to embark on concentrated research regarding naturopathic cures for all ailments and issues. I particularly pride the joyful experience of avoiding any medical intervention during the phases of menopause. My friends warned me of the HRT, surgical procedures and discomforts that were inevitable. Certainly, I had some symptoms and my family were very tolerant of my mood swings, but it did not last very long. A year later, I was free! Similarly, all members of my family are learning how to avoid disease or cure it naturally at its early stages. Those diseases which remain, are due to some weakness in discipline or knowledge and we are aware that we need to keep learning so that we can manage our mental health issues.

## Healthy Eating Habits

There are many sources of guidance regarding the medicinal benefits of food and also how it is prepared and consumed. In Ayurvedic medicine, each food source has a specific quantity and time for consumption. Many dietitians advise the various types of diet. The Keto diet, the alkali diet, the high protein diet and many more.

**Fasting.** A Muslim is expected to fast for one month a year in Ramadhan. Every religion has prescribed fasting. Fasting has also become a popular method of weight-loss. The purpose of fasting is to regulate behaviour and appetite. As I discussed earlier, there are many benefits to fasting. Fasting enables us to clean out the digestive system. If we eat to fill our stomach, then we have restricted space for the digesting process. Many toxins collect in the digestive tracts and need a clean-up. The acts of fasting and also the act of leaving some space in our stomach and not over-eating can ensure that we keep our digestive system clean.

The **"American Diet"** is considered the most acceptable in social settings and so it is a social challenge to consume in a healthy manner. Children are the most innocent victims of the "American diet" consisting of pizzas and burgers and cookies, all over the world. This is how they become "comfort foods" and this is a difficult habit to break. Food is processed and water is replaced with pop or shakes. The body battles with this stressful habit. It is a challenge to very young stomachs.

In a depressed state, it is natural to eat what is nearby and prepared. That huge bag of chips in the kitchen is very tempting. When anxious or depressed, in the fight or flight state, it is natural to eat whatever is available. This is more the case if these are the "comfort foods". If the anxiety triggers are predictable, then to anticipate that, it is good to keep a store of healthy snacks in the fridge to provide good nutrition in those anxious or down times. Yellow coloured fruits and veggies are known to have happy hormones and a happy affect. Pineapple, bananas, yellow peppers and sweetcorn work well. It is possible to train the brain to go for these foods at those times so that they become the comfort foods.

**Prayer Before Eating**. As a believer, I would also include prayer in my food preparation and consumption. Since I have made it a habit that I pray for Allah's blessing as I add each ingredient, I feel more alert and confident about what I am preparing and the nutritional value of each ingredient. I am also more grateful for the benefits of each ingredient. Before a meal, I pray;

*In the name of Allah and with the blessings of Allah.*

## Water Consumption.

One more aspect which I should really have mentioned first, is our consumption of clean water. We installed a filter and ensured that we maintained good hygiene, however we were not consuming enough water. Water is the first source of nourishment for a baby and without it we would die. So, Allah has created within us a strong force of thirst. If we are extremely thirsty we develop a headache in the top of our head. We must address thirst seriously in order to enable the other nutrients to be transported to all needy parts of the body. The Holy Prophet of Islam taught us that giving water to the thirsty is a great act of charity. He taught us that it is the first thing we should consume when breaking a fast. He taught us to sip water slowly three sips at a time when we drink. He taught us to drink while sitting down. He also taught us that if we are angry, we must drink water to cool our nerves. Allah has blessed us with basic knowledge of survival. One young lady suffering from acute depression realised that her symptoms were worse when she was dehydrated. With the constant reminders from family and friends, she increased her consumption and her awareness that when she has a depressive episode she should first sit down and drink a good amount of fresh water. Often, that was all she needed to overcome her depressive state and so she did not need to take her extra, emergency pill. In the journaling section of this book, you will be reflecting on your water consumption.

## 2.Quality Sleep

The market for sleep management and relaxation has boomed in the past 20 years. There are DVDs, CDs, apps, YouTube videos and many workshops which you can attend to learn how to sleep. I find that very amusing. Our lifestyle has made us nocturnal. In Islam, we are expected to sleep after the night prayer and wake early for the morning prayer. The market for meditation has also boomed. CEOs and business gurus are all investing in meditation classes and products to increase their productivity and quality of life. In the journaling section of this book, you will be reflecting on these aspects of your life.

## 3.Positive Social interaction

So, I eat well and I sleep better, but how do I cope with all the negative energy of society? Earlier, I mentioned the list of ways to stay socially active. In the journaling section of this book, you will be reflecting on these aspects of your life;

**1.Visit a friend**. If I visit a friend who is feeling down herself then our meeting will involve indulging in our sorrows and encouraging hopelessness. If I am in a down mood, then I need to decide to visit someone in a positive mood and plan to do something fun or constructive together. In my local community, each department of the organization is kept busy and there is a department to cater for every skill and interest. We are always helping someone in a very charitable manner.

**2.Visit a place of worship or community centre**. If I attend a community event, it needs to be one which will uplift me. In my community, it is very difficult to motivate members to attend events of an academic nature. The attendance to practical or fun events is much more inviting. So, now there is an increasing number of events which are interactive and meaningful to the practical lives of members.

**3.Go shopping.** The shopping experience liberates the creative mind. It allows the mind to indulge in positive criticism and appreciate the beautiful creations of others. The shopping experience can be an exciting social experience whereby you can connect with your companion in new ways learning and appreciating their likes and dislikes. If it is not enjoyable, it can be a financially dangerous activity. I do not like window shopping. I like to make a list, research where I can get the best deal and then just go and buy the items. I am not keen on online shopping because of the probability of having to return half of what I buy.

**4.Play a sport or games.** There is a sport for all types of people. If you know what your skills are and have friends who share those skills, then there is a sport for you. Unfortunately, it may be expensive to play the sport of choice and so you may need to compromise. Many like to play computer games. I like to play board games with my family. My experience of sports is limited due to asthma and glasses when I was a child. My ability to aim has always been embarrassing, so I avoided many sports activities. I only play sports that I have a chance to be competitive. The key is to be challenged in a fun way to take the mind off the mundane stresses of daily life. I like to remind my family that "family that plays, prays and eats together, stays together" So, we enjoy most activities together; even cleaning and cooking.

*And everyone has a goal which dominates him; vie, then, with one another in good works. Wherever you be, Allah will bring you all together. Surely, Allah has the power to do all that He wills.* CH2 Verse 149

This, surely generates a good supply of serotonin.

**5.Work-out at a Gym.** A few years ago, we owned a Gym. My husband had opened a Gym business, and members enjoyed working out and meeting each other. They often popped their head into the office to chat with my husband who loved to encourage them to achieve their goals. We would also go once a week to the Gym to work out. After we sold the Gym, my husband and son ingeniously converted the garage into a Gym for the family. This worked out to be a very convenient way of supplementing our endorphins to keep ourselves in a positive mindset. It also ensured a regular fitness routine with no excuses that we cannot get to a Gym. If I did not have this facility, I would certainly join any local gym or find a part of my home to engage in a suitable workout routine.

**6.Walk in a Park or an Open Space.** My family have made a habit of walking around the local park after dinner in the summer and the mall in the colder months. A brisk walk in any season is a sure way to freshen our body and clear the mind. The action of changing location for a while and getting some fresh air is the best fight against any type of depression. However, it is when you are in a depressed state that you do not feel like getting ready and going out. As I mentioned before, it is a struggle unless it is a routine by which you will meet others. As a Muslim, I can walk to the mosque five times a day. I remember as a child that a Muslim neighbour in London, UK, and my father's good friend, left his front door open since there was always someone coming in and out of the house and he himself was retired, so he walked 20 minutes to the mosque for each prayer, every day. He was a very happy and stress-free man, all his children were leading citizens, and his wife was very patient and hard-working.

There are many benefits to going out in the sun. Most of all, it is the best way to generate vitamin D, which is essential for the immune system to fight disease, for bone health and to be happy. That great feeling of sunshine on your face and eyes is heaped in health benefits and happiness. Dressing modestly, with a hijab is no excuse. If your face gets some sun, that is good enough.

**7.Get a Physically Challenging Job.** The Holy Prophet of Islam also promoted actively earning one's living and running the home independently. Laziness is frowned upon. Modern society is suffering from unemployment and the ideal that employment is only for the purpose of making or saving money, for financial success. However, for many, their job is a social respite. If the job is also physically challenging, then you get your workout as well. Some jobs require you to sit for hours, so, some companies reward their staff for joining the Gym. Many people are extremely challenged financially and work 7 days with two jobs. This is the other extreme and needs to be addressed to avoid burn-out.

As a teacher, I have seen an increase in childhood complaints of being tired, having aches and pains and behavioural issues. I believe, there is a relationship between this and the increased use of technology. How will these children be able to work a full day and manage their family life? To build stamina, the adults need to model healthy physical activity and a healthy lifestyle. Most Gyms only allow adults over 13years, so in their leisure time the parents are away from their children. Family sports and fitness activities would keep the whole family fit and happy together. As a bonus, the family collects a healthy amount of happy memories. If adults can model an enjoyment of hard work and busyness, the children learn to be hard-working and resilient. If parents are working late shifts for 7 days a week, then children can be encouraged to learn to support the family with chores. This is also a good way to generate endorphins and dopamine in the body.

**8.Pursue a Hobby.** Society is so heavily financially challenged now, that it is hard to imagine a hobby. However, any hobby is a healthy distraction from the stresses of life and can open new doors of social activity which is creative or interesting. A change is always as good as a rest. My hobby was singing. Singing is a therapeutic cure for whole body function. As a child, I always loved singing at school and realised my musical mind. Music and singing are a motivation for me. So, I joined the school choir and the mosque singing groups. This hobby developed my social skills as well as strengthening my heart and digestive system.

## 4.Exercise.

This is an aspect of our lifestyle which we usually remember on New Year's Day. We look in the mirror and frown at how we squeezed that body into the party outfits we wore during the holiday week. How many of us covered it up with a cardigan or jacket? But it is still there and it can give us a very miserable start to the new year. The weather in the northern hemisphere is dull and gloomy, we are feeling overindulged and probably regret some conversation we had over the holiday week and then we look at this body. So, we make a resolution and charts and pay for Gym membership with our credit card on our laptop lying in bed and order Gym clothes from the online sale and perhaps we order a Gym machine to put in the game room in our home so we don't need to go to a Gym. In the journaling section of this book, you will be reflecting on these aspects of your fitness.

Have we really found a solution to our endorphin drain? Probably not. The key is to get out of the house and start an activity which yields a result. Sports, gardening, coaching, a new more active job, taking public transport to work, cycling to work. All of these activities can and must be continued and can sustain a healthy exercise routine. Our ancestors would walk miles to post a letter or sell goods at a market, or even collect water for daily use. I could discuss various exercises, but the truth is that even though we ran a Gym and have one in the garage, the best exercise my family have sustained are the commute to school or work and a long shopping trip to the mall or grocery shopping.

# STEP 3: SOCIAL AND EMOTIONAL HEALTH.

## Personal Identity

Although, this chapter is intended to enable us to face society with confidence, the most essential power in the success of a society is the emotional wellbeing of individuals who constitute the society. If my personal identity is dependent on my role in society, then I am not yet whole. I need to understand myself as a personality. For that, I need to reflect on the talents which Allah has gifted me as well as the lessons which I have learned from my life experiences. For this, I need to be mindful. I need to be aware of my emotions. I need to address my emotions and control them so that my learning experience is positive and enables me to grow. I need to assess my own biases and prejudices and my ability to communicate effectively. In the journaling section of this book, you will be reflecting on these aspects of your personality.

I have learned in my professional practice to control my emotions and sometimes suppress them so that I am able to deescalate a situation with an upset student in a primary classroom. I had mastered this ability to such a level, that I applied the same behaviours with my own children. As they grew, I realised that my inability to expose my true emotions had created an emotional wall around me and I had modelled for my children that one must suppress true emotions. I felt that they were learning to be resilient. Unfortunately, they learned to distance themselves from me and to hide their true feelings. When they grew older, they started to open up with their father and he was able to understand their true emotions and communicate them to me. Gradually, I learned to express my own true emotions and as a result, we all started to experience true happiness and genuine love. By addressing our true emotions, we are able to understand our identity, our core values and our true desires. Once this is activated, we are able to understand who we can connect with and how we can communicate with the universal language of love and friendship.

We are all realising that racism is actually a distraction which obstructs us from positive social interaction and growth. By addressing racism and all the other isms, we are able to open doors of communication and are able to learn from all the humans Allah has created, in a positive way. Rather than wasting half of every day explaining why I wear hijab, eat halal food, pray and fast in Ramadhan, I am able to have a meaningful conversation with my colleagues and friends in any social setting about issues which excite my personality. I can connect with people who share my passions and inspirations. I can build true and lasting relationships with my chosen husband and family and friends and my children. I reduce my fear of boredom, failure, embarrassment, and many other aspects of fear and grief.

## My Name

When people talk to me, the first intriguing aspect is my name. I am ethnic Pakistani but my name is Irish. My mother will explain. I struggled with my personality as a child. I felt like Sheila but looked like Zahida. Having to explain is annoying. I have a good friend who is ethnic Italian but her parents changed her name to a more Canadian one for the same reason. I am at peace with both my names now but it took some personal growth to get there. I urge you all to value your name and never compromise its pronunciation. Students are always delighted when I pronounce their name correctly. This is the truth about you. On the first day of school I would ensure that the teacher understood how to pronounce my children's names.

The Holy Prophet of Islam said;

*"Truth saves, falsehood destroys"*

By being honest with myself and expressing and embracing my true emotions, I gain the power to be creative rather than destructive. How exciting would it be if people took the time to text themselves and chat with themselves instead of texting others to see how many likes and responses they get. If everyone could truly say; "I liked myself 700 times today", the resulting joy would generate a magnetic smile, radiating joy everywhere. So, the aim is to be comfortable with our personal identity and communicate this in social settings so that we are surrounded by like-minded people, including our family. Since it is very difficult to identify that in others, the process of finding the right life-partner is better left to Allah. I will discuss this later.

## Intimate Relationships

As adults, one aspect of our lives which some term as taboo is our sexuality. Contemporary society is plagued with an obsession with sexuality which crept into the world of media, lifting the veil of modesty and has exploited this obsession in all spheres of society. I found it really very awkward when my teenage son casually talked to me about male and female electronic connections. Is it really necessary to call them that?

A solution, provided by Islam, which has been lost in many other societies but has so greatly disturbed the status quo that some governments have passed laws banning it is the veil for men and women. Allah explains the concept of chastity. He explains that men and women must control their carnal desires out of wedlock. If we consider honestly, what we are most fearful of, it is usually related to relationships, and our desire is to have an exclusive, pure relationship by which we can set up a family. Children have always loved stories of a prince and princess who get married and live "happily ever after". Prophet Muhammad (peace be upon him) advised; "Truth saves, falsehood destroys" By hiding the truth of human relations, society is destroying itself and the media is the most aggressive weapon against chastity.

The Holy Quran defines chastity in CH24 verse 31 to 32;

*Say to the believing men that they restrain their eyes and guard their private parts. That is purer for them. Surely, Allah is well aware of what they do.*
*And say to the believing women that they restrain their eyes and guard their private parts, and that they disclose not their natural and artificial beauty except that which is apparent thereof, and that they draw their head-coverings over their bosoms, and that they disclose not their beauty save to their husbands, or to their fathers, or the fathers of their husbands or their sons or the sons of their husbands or their brothers, or the sons of their brothers, or the sons of their sisters, or their women, or what their right hands possess, or such of male attendants as have no sexual appetite, or young children who have no knowledge of the hidden parts of women. And they strike not their feet so that what they hide of their ornaments may become known. And turn ye to Allah all together, O believers, that you may succeed.*

Society has breached all of these aspects so completely that there seems to be no hope for future generations to find true chastity again. We yearn for true, trusting and loving relationships but they are as rare as truly organic food. These rules are to safeguard the eyes and ears of men and women from the attraction of men and women whom they are not legally related to. Being legally related ensures the responsibility of taking care of the relationship and their dependants. To assist men in their efforts to maintain their chastity, women are required to hide their beauty behind a veil and to walk gently so that they do not distract men. The media encourages women to dress immodestly and to wear heels and stamp their feet as they walk to impose their power over men. It is very challenging to find modest clothing in regular retail stores. Almost all items have extra holes somewhere to reveal some part of the body and entice men. If we consider each element of the instruction in the Holy Quran;

**1.Restrain The Eyes.** Unfortunately, modern cultures require that conversations maintain eye-contact. The eyes are the window to the heart. By maintaining eye-contact, it can be very easy to realise if there is an attraction. In addition, modern culture requires that men and women shake hands. The chemical exchange by shaking hands can seal the deal for some and hence the fantasy can continue in the minds of both and cause some harm to existing legal relationships or future relationships. I have watched my friends and colleagues dating. This remedy cannot be ignored. It is a powerful remedy.

**2.Restrain The Ears.** Although the verse refers to the sound of women walking, there are many more ways now to distract the ears. The media has normalised pop music to such a level that, now, children will not engage in silent reading at school without headphones. It seems we cannot do anything without pop music. When I challenged my children to listen carefully to lyrics, it transformed their taste in music. However, I could not stop them from listening to music because everyone around them had the habit as well. I am very selective in what I listen to but I do like to listen in my car. The issue is that I am listening to men and women singing. These songs do influence my mood and my thinking. My playlist is a very positive one. At school and in malls and in movies and everywhere else, we are at the mercy of the society we live in.

**3.Restrain Ears From Descriptions.** As a teacher, I often hear boys and girls describing each other or celebrities as beautiful, but then also quite immodest and sometimes shameless terms are used. This is a painful experience for those who are being described and for those who have respect for the personalities being described.

**4.Restrain Relationships.** Society has made dating a cultural norm for many. If dating can be avoided, and relationships may be taken more seriously, then adults may be more responsible. It is exacerbated by the abuse of contraceptives. Adults have been provided an opportunity to hide their adultery so they can take any relationship to its end without any commitment for the future. The result is a high proportion of single parent families whereby mothers are trying to be mother and father while the men continue to have multiple love-less relationships and eventually become mentally ill as well.

**Finding The Right Life-Partner**

A Muslim is advised that he or she should carefully consider the criteria for his or her life partner. One may marry for good looks, wealth, status or piety. Priority should be given to piety since that is what sustains a happy marriage.

When looking for a life-partner, there are so many fears attached with making the right decision. Again, if we consider that Allah has our blueprint, then it is logical that Allah also knows who we are compatible with. At the time when I had to make this decision, I left the decision entirely to Allah. He showed me in many related dreams and indications that I should marry and stay married to my husband. The reason I enjoyed this experience was because I engaged in a special prayer for decision making. The *istekhaara* prayer is for all major decisions whereby I ask Allah if the project (such as marriage) is right for me then make it happen easily and if not then take it away from me and replace it with the right one according to Allah's decree.

*O Allah, I seek good from Thee out of Thy knowledge and seek power from Thee out of Thy power and I beg of Thee out of Thy boundless Grace, for Thou hast power and I have no power, and Thou hast knowledge and I have no knowledge, and Thy knowledge encompasses the unseen.*

*O Allah! If it be within Thy knowledge that this task is for my good, both materially and spiritually, and in respect of my ultimate end, then make it possible for me and bless me therein, but if it be within Thy knowledge that it is harmful for me in my spiritual and material life and in respect of my ultimate end, then turn me away therefrom, and enable me to attain good wherever it may be and cause me to be blessed therewith.*

The response to this prayer is expected as a dream, an unexpected occurrence, or indication or a deep satisfaction that one should continue with the project. This whole process is deeply satisfying and removes all sense of fear or regret. I use this prayer for all my projects and for my children as well. Some people ask others to pray for them. This is only because they are not confident in their relationship with Allah. I advise them to reflect on how much they trust Allah and then pray for themselves.

## The Family Unit

Trust is necessary for any relationship to work. Trust requires the courage to tell the whole truth and face the consequences. Trust also requires a willingness to listen carefully with compassion and to express a desire to forgive. After many years of observing and helping friends and family, I have become aware that women are mostly in fear of the husband leaving them. I would say the number one fear of humans is the fear of rejection. So, we conform. This can hinder the opportunity to thrive. In Islam, men and women are permitted divorce and men are also permitted up to four wives. Islam has had a bad press regarding these two allowances. The media has missed some very important conditions attached to them.

When they become parents, the couple have a firm standing on the foundations of a healthy and happy childhood for their children. They are able to facilitate the learning of pious character traits and etiquettes that will ensure their children are respectful to society and the environment. I ensure that there is a physical or at least an emotional veil between me and men who I am not related to. I abstain from free mixing in social gatherings and I have devoted my life and love to my husband and our family.

The ideas presented earlier can be applied to family life and the parents can launch healthy habits. I have found that parents fear the futures for their children because there is some malfunction in the family unit. Some mothers tell me that the communication and understanding between the parents is so poor that they cannot agree on many issues. I have worked closely with a family which was at the brink of separation. The key here was trust. There are many Muslims who are not able to sustain a marriage and for allowable reasons, they may divorce. Often the reason is miscommunication and misunderstandings. This results from the habit of ignoring the truth and acting on cultural or personal biases and expectations. In the journaling section of this book, you have the opportunity to examine your own biases and how they influence your decisions.

## Avoiding Divorce

Divorce is permitted in Islam. Internationally, divorce is a legal procedure. When a couple engages a lawyer, they have completed the discussion and there is only a very remote chance of reconciliation. The court proceedings are a formality to ensure that financial affairs and the child custody issues are legally settled. Divorce is permitted in Islam if there is any cheating in the relationship or the couple have become completely incompatible due to a breakdown in communication. However, as I mentioned, this communication breakdown may be due to some behaviors related to outside pressures, biases or even mental illness. The breakdown may stem from the inability to forgive and show compassion. It is possible that if the husband or wife alone concentrate their effort to focus on the thinking and mental health of the family, then the matters can be resolved. It takes much bravery to do it, but it is possible.

One example is a man who became very sick. He became so ill that he resigned from work and decided to treat himself. He also decided that he could not cope with his family. He isolated himself at home and nearly every month a petty disagreement gave him the excuse for divorce. Deep down in his mind, he seemed to have decided that being incurable, he would just live for himself, since he did not want to argue with his family. The wife knew that, in fact it was a lifetime of low self-esteem and trust issues which had made him sick and he needed to address his mental health first. The wife started adding herbs and foods to the diet to calm the anxiety, and provide nutrients for brain health and strength. She avoided any confrontations. Any time he threatened to leave, she allowed him to plan that and allowed him to plan to live apart. He never did leave and after a few days he would settle again. Her key was that she prayed for him all day and, more importantly, she also focussed on her own behaviour and character traits to address her personality honestly. She realised that compassion and cooperation was the cure for their issues. She also realised that her husband's episodes coincided with her menstrual cycle and he was being affected by her hormones. She could predict those days and prevent conflict. She also realised that she herself was in denial of some mental health issues of her own. They dedicated their time to their relationship and the children were also encouraged to learn to forgive and to enjoy their company and to share their lives with them honestly and openly. Gradually, he became more involved in his family and the children and the wife started sharing the truth of their feelings and emotions of their lives. This family has learned to enjoy every moment and many new prayers and activities together. Most of all, the family learned to laugh away their problems with some help from the herbs and foods and prayers and to give quality time to discuss any issues carefully.

There are many etiquettes and routines that can improve the quality of family life. Family meal time can be a daily practice. We pray before we eat, out of gratitude for the food and the person who prepared or provided it. Family can pray together, play together, make meals together, go out together, exercise together, and even have sleepovers together in the living room! It is the efforts of both parents that keep a family together. If money is tight, then lower the family budget and demands. Learn skills together so that family members can create and mend household needs and save money. Our best friend is *GOOGLE*. If we need to fix or make something, we 'Google' it and then attempt to fix it together. It can be so much fun. Much more fun that buying the replacement online or in the shops and then struggle with the resulting financial burden.

So, what aspects of family life can cause fear or grief? Family relationships can be impacted in many ways, some unimaginable. Strained relationships due to existing mental health issues stemmed from past experiences can show themselves as low self-esteem, inferiority complex, trust issues and some somatic illnesses. Extensive family conflicts which have escalated over time and become too elaborate to solve such as disputes over inheritance or favoritism.

Poor conflict-resolution skills can leave issues hanging unsolved and as they pile up can cause a domino effect when it becomes overwhelming. Poor family communication patterns such as passive-aggressive reactions, or silence. This is exacerbated by the negative biases promoted in the family such as;

**a. Resistance to change.** "This is how we have always viewed things in our culture"
**b. View of others.** "This is how we have always been perceived."
**c. Rigidity of rules.** "These are the unbreakable rules of our society".

All of this is modelled by all members of the family. This can lead to insecurity and depression. It takes a lot of courage to break the mould. This is necessary to overcome the grief of inadequate relationships.

## Cultural Norms

Society enforces unnecessary rules on us which limit us in every sphere of our lives. The only way to grow our own mind is to liberate ourselves from the unnecessary rules. In Islam there are more than 700 rules and injunctions in the Holy Quran. I understand them all, but I do not know if there is anyone who is following all of them, all the time. Those rules are there to guide us onto the righteous path. Every day in our prayers, we ask Allah to guide us on the right path. Even prophets of all religions and religious leaders ask Allah to guide them onto the right path. There is no prayer in Islam in which we ask Allah to make us *perfect*. Allah says in the Holy Quran that Islam is the perfect religion. However, we also know that only Allah is perfect and that is what defines Allah the Creator. Allah tells us to pray for forgiveness every day and to read the Holy Quran every day with reflection and understanding. By following this daily routine, we gain ownership of our learning and we adopt the rules necessary for us in our own lives. Through our lives, we focus on one rule after another developing our personality and character traits which take us to the wisdom of elderly life. This is how we are able to model healthy behaviours for the next generation.

## Bias

Cultural norms are based on bias. On reflection, we all have bias towards attitudes. Our bias can affect our mental health as well as the mental health of those we interact with. We may have a bias regarding beauty, wealth, health, ability or disabilities which are all exhibited in our behaviours. These biases are congruent with our values and are developed from childhood. Facing new people or social settings, cause an inner conflict whereby we are making judgements in order to decide how we will behave. Consider the first day at a new workplace. Entering the building, your bias and core values enable you to judge the level of management and you are already subconsciously adjusting yourself and realising how you may fit in with the culture of this workplace. You have made many judgements before meeting any staff members. For some aspects you may feel shame that you are inadequate for that setting. You may feel confused and this can lead to unnecessary stress stemming from the fear of inadequacy. You may even recall your previous workplace and feel grief at the loss of that job. In this short time, you have decided if you will be successful and even how you will greet the first person you meet.

If you are not familiar with the concept of bias, just consider how you choose a new friend. What is it that attracts you? Do you believe that tall people are beautiful and successful and powerful? Have you never met a powerful person who is short? Do you believe that children with special educational needs will not be able to pursue a profession? Have you never met a genius who has autism? These biases exist in our minds and we judge others and ourselves by them. These judgements can make us weak and hinder our success.

# STEP 4: BANKING MEMORIES

## Memories

Childhood memories are very powerful. As a parent and parent counselor, I have focussed on building positive memories. Babies need to be loved and parents enjoy that time with their children. As the child becomes independent in its play and actions, parents begin to detach themselves and have less interaction until it becomes a mundane routine of breakfast, sign letters and agenda, depart for school, after-school care, homework, dinner and bedtime. Weekends are family chores and movies or surfing the internet and texting or being with friends and then Monday returns. The family waits for the holidays to make the memories. This is the standard contemporary family routine. Reflecting on my childhood, my fondest childhood memories are watching my mother, carefully colouring my volcano picture, going to our local library with my mother, gardening with my parents, having fascinating discussions with my father at the Science Museum in London every Sunday while eating horse chestnuts from the stall outside where we parked the car. I remember playing cricket with my brother in our bedroom with our soft toys and the mini cricket bat my father made for them. I had a lovely childhood. I learned that my parents loved me and believed in me and my brother and valued our interests. They provided and compensated for our needs. I do also remember how we budgeted as a family and how important hospitality and compassion for guests was.

Everyone has good memories with someone. My memories of negative events are very weak because my parents showed me how to solve problems and forgive. In my childhood there were many very challenging negative events and I do have some disturbing memories, but my strongest memories for them are how we overcame them because I learned to have a growth mindset from my parents. If you reflect on your memories, then you can see clearly how you developed your personality. If you focus on the negative memories, you develop some negative personality traits. If you focus on some of the positive memories, you develop positive personality traits. The aim is to create enough positive memories to generate a majority positive government in your heart. When you face a challenge, the majority vote is to see the positive side of the challenge and solve the problem and then to grow from it. This, again is the true meaning of

*Jihad*. At this point, I would recommend the activity to make a list of positive and negative memories and understand how you have learned from it. In the journaling section of this book, you will be reflecting on these aspects of your memories.

## Actions and Emotions

As a teacher, it is my goal to enable my students to take powerful action to meet the needs of their emotions. I aim to facilitate learning by generating excitement for that learning. I am always aware that children bring other emotions to school every day which are reflections of what they have experienced outside of the classroom. These are sometimes termed as Adverse Childhood Experiences. Many of these experiences are due to adult experiences and are witnessed by children. These are the detrimental experiences which create the negative memories which are carried into adulthood. In Islam, we are advised to learn to forgive and in our daily prayers we ask Allah to forgive our parents and accept their prayers. In my experience of contemporary counselling techniques, it is only recently that patients are being encouraged to forgive. Some practitioners are asserting that the act of forgiveness may even be the cure for some diseases. I have seen that in many cases.

### Forgive.

In order to forgive, one must be able to address the emotions involved in the event. It is very easy to blame our mental state on an event or a person without considering why that event occurred or how that person was at the time. The most powerful action to launch healing, is to forgive. In the Muslim prayer, we first ask Allah to forgive us and then to forgive others. The prayers for forgiveness are given great importance. An event may cause a lot of stress at the time, but that stress increases exponentially for as long as we hold on to it. No amount of stress relieving medication will be as powerful as the act of letting it go by the act of forgiving.

On many occasions, I have been tested in this way. On one occasion, I was involved in a very important project. I had put all my effort into this and my heart was so engaged in it that I did not realise how I was neglecting my other needs. I believed in this project. Due to a misunderstanding, my work on the project ended abruptly. Friends and strangers asked me why I was no longer involved. I felt guilty and betrayed. My feelings escalated as the days, months and years filled with constant reminders of the project and my memories of events during the project. I became quite dejected. I wanted reassurance that I was forgiven and I also needed to forgive so that it could end and I could move on. Over time, the negative memories were replaced with positive memories. I met members of the team and became more relaxed about talking about the project. Eventually, I was at peace because the process of forgiveness was complete. The feelings of fear and grief were so heavy that I could have become very seriously ill, but because I was surrounded by like-minded, positive friends and family, I was able to experience the process of forgiveness completely.

*Tell those who believe to forgive those who persecute them and fear not the Days of Allah, that He may requite a people for what they earn.* CH45 Verse15

This whole process requires a growth mindset. This step requires that we plan to learn from negative experiences and reject the desire for revenge. If society can realise that all humans have the capacity for love and forgiveness, then it would be a healthier society. Hate, crimes, war and injustice all stem from the inability to forgive or show compassion. As such, Islam requires two steps in the forgiveness process.

1.*Istaghfar.* To ask Allah to cover our sins for us and forgive us. This step is an agreement with Allah that we recognise that we have wronged our soul by committing the sin. *Istaghfar* is fuelled by strength.

*And whoso does evil or wrongs his soul, and then asks forgiveness of Allah, will surely find Allah Most Forgiving, Merciful.* CH4 Verse111

2.*Taubah.* To repent to Allah for help to never commit that sin again out of a genuine feeling of remorse. Taubah is fuelled by resolve.

*And He it is Who accepts repentance from His servants, and forgives sins. And He knows what you do.* Ch42 Verse 26

Both steps are fuelled with positive energy and strength and certainly are pleasing to Allah. That is how He can efface our sins. In the journaling section of this book, you will have the opportunity to try a traffic lights system for solving problems and achieving a solution and hence forgiveness.

# STEP 5: EMOTIONAL HABITS

There are so many different kinds of emotions which correspond to the attributes of Allah. We learn to engage these emotions as very young children when it is modelled by the adults on whom we depend for guidance. Quite simply, the reason I love children is because my mother loved children. My love for children was also encouraged by my middle school experience and my religious education teacher who always reminded us that Jesus (peace be upon him) said that "The Kingdom of Heaven is for children"

*Jesus said, "Let the little children come to me, and do not hinder them, for the kingdom of heaven belongs to such as these."* Bible Matt 19:14

I think I decided then, that I did not want to be a serious adult and I would stay with children as long as I could. However, that attitude did stall my attempts to address my emotions. This is something I learned later in life.

It is vital to address emotions properly and respectfully. By synchronizing our thoughts and emotions, we are enabled to achieve pure levels of creative energy and solve problems and then grow from the experience. I have only recently taken the time to address emotions. I had ignored them as a weakness before. If, instead, we consider the powerful energy of our emotions, then we are able to channel that energy to heal and solve issues from the present and even past experiences. These powerful emotions are stored in our subconscious. Such a waste! When I started to address my emotions and pull them out of my subconscious and literally write them down in my journal, I realized just how immensely powerful they are.

## The Power of Negative Emotions

### Anger

Anger teaches us about how assertive and inflexible we are. Anger displays a clear message of suppression and a weak ability to show compassion. We show anger when we feel that someone has violated our rights or our values or rules or our needs.

### Sadness

Sadness is an expression of the need for compassion. Sadness conveys the message that I am alone and unsupported. I need someone to connect with me and listen to me and address my needs.

## Grief

The loss of something important leads to grief. The level of grief is an indication of how strong our bond and dependence is with the object or the personality and how resilient we are. An awareness of our level of resilience is vital to recovery from any mental illness.

## Anxiety

Our level of anxiety when we face a challenge is a clear indication of our resilience but also is a clear indicator of what issues are most important to us. Anxiety is strongly linked to fear since we become anxious when we fear an outcome or we fear the consequences of expressing our true feelings.

## Frustration

Frustration is caused by impatience. Impatience is the result of a weakness in compassion. Frustration leads to anger and can lead to anxiety. Frustration is also an indication of our level of perfectionism. We have set a standard and if it is not achieved perfectly then we may become frustrated.

All of these and many other negative emotions indicate clearly that it is very important to address our emotions honestly to avoid destruction. I refer again to the simple but powerful saying of Prophet Muhammad (peace be upon him). "Truth saves, falsehood destroys". Not addressing these emotions can result in behaviours which can create a negative wall around your true intentions and can destructively escalate the negativity.

We need to make how we appear due to our actions coherent with how we really are with our true intentions. Prophet Muhammad (peace be upon him) once said that: "Actions are judged by intentions" Teasing out this saying reveals that society cannot forgive us if we cannot express our intentions properly in our actions. We need to be patient with ourselves and our emotions. If we take time to address how we feel and how we are motivated, then we can engage in our actions with true intentions and achieve our goal. Technology in our hands, have made society spontaneous in actions. I often meet people who grieve about a consequence of a regrettable text message or action. Children are learning that there are quick ways to get answers to even emotional questions. You can Google "why does my mom yell at me when I don't wake up" Mom has made a habit of not addressing emotions, so the child needs to find the answer himself in order to address his emotion. If mom could say "I am getting late for work and I need to know that you will get on the school bus and take your lunch, please can you get up now", son knows which emotion is involved in her yelling. As well as our brief communications, we have vague texts and accompanying emojis. These habits are causing us to neglect our emotions and resulting in dangerous life decisions. We simply need to give more time to our thoughts and reflect on what we truly want for ourselves. Society claims to be liberated and individualist but, in reality, it appears to be like a herd of sheep following leaders blindly. Society does not seem to have time for reflection and thought. Life is described to be a race whereby everyone is struggling to gather as much material as possible before death takes them away. The world is littered with unclaimed belongings since there are few sentiments and memories attached to them. Just imagine how many memories, sentiments and emotions are lost in a garage sale.

## The Power of Positive Emotions

Educators speak of resilience training for children. Why do educators now need to teach children to be resilient? Why is this training being meted out to other members of the village that raises each child? I believe that society has devalued the role of parents and extended family.

### Love

The most powerful emotion which nurtures resilience is love. True love from parents, siblings and extended family members provides an inner strength to each child. Love is the most powerful and essential emotion. Where there is love, there is growth and learning. Love fuels passion. Passion fuels creativity and creativity fuels life.

In my childhood, the word love became a taboo since in England at that time, love was mostly associated with lust. However, there was so much love in my family and so much passion and creativity that I learned to search for love in everything.

### Trust

Love is fueled by trust. Where there is trust, there is gratitude and love. Trust is an inner emotion and action. Trust can be broken easily but can also be regained through open and honest communication. Trust is fueled by honesty and courage.

## Courage

Courage requires an ability to trust one's conviction. If you are able to trust your own values and emotions and are ready fight for your beliefs, your love, your case or your cause, then you have the power of courage.

By conquering all of these emotions, we are able to become fearless and faithful. These powerful emotions can change the life of the anxious mind. A believer is armed with the ability to accept all of these emotions and that is why Allah says that a believer will not fear or grieve. We can only be the best of who we are in our various roles in order to be accomplished. We need to be in control of these emotions. I have applied this idea to my Islamic lifestyle and feel a closeness to Allah that empowers me to engage in these and many other positive emotions.

When I realised that I was not in control, I addressed how I love and trust people, I realised that I was blindly obedient. Blind obedience can be useful in an organised community but, after a while, it can create feelings of resentment and lower self-esteem. The passion with which one launches into an activity can fade over time since there is a weakness in the level of honesty, trust and equity. Obedience is a positive action in a trusting, equitable relationship which is based on mutual respect. I realised that respect is earned through positive actions and honest, courageous actions. I needed to feel that my coworkers trust me and share my values.

As a Muslim, I am required to obey Allah. However, Allah has also instructed me to reflect and find understanding in my readings of His book of instructions. Allah does not want blind obedience, He wants me to understand His rules and follow them with passion, courage and trust. When I apply that to my daily interactions at work and home and on the road, I realise that I am consciously obedient rather than blindly obedient. Consider driving on the road. When approaching an amber light, we should slow down and consider if we should continue or stop. The rule requires us to reflect and show understanding. If we clearly see that the road is clear and there are no vehicles or pedestrians, then we may cross the amber light. If it is a busy road and many pedestrians and traffic, then we must consider stopping at amber in case there is a need. If we are waiting to turn into a side road at the lights but oncoming traffic is heavy, then we may wait for the amber light, in order to turn since that is the only opportunity when we trust that the oncoming traffic may slow down or stop. As a believer, we are required to consider others and their needs all the time. There are many occasions when we may need to be flexible with rules and forgive others. We need to trust others and understand their intentions.

The scenarios described require many positive emotions. These emotions have the ability to prevent misunderstandings and destructive, negative emotions. If we are able to understand our emotions, then we can empower ourselves with the ability to manage fear and grief in a respectful way. This is our goal. My goal is to find love in everyone. However, it is a very high goal for which we all strive in our *jihad* to reach.

# STEP 6: REFLECT AND SELF-REFORM

Considering all of what I have learned, in my life journey, the most powerful activity in my life is the act of reflecting and trying to self-reform and grow. I have journaled in many ways and have grown each time. I have kept diaries, journals, written articles, written poems and had many discussions at home and with groups of children, youth and adults. I have realised that this is the true purpose in life. This is how we worship Allah. A powerful action is the act of gratitude. I can never thank my Creator enough for all the amazing experiences He has provided me to learn about who I am and why I am. I have enjoyed all my experiences, even the negative experiences. I am eternally grateful for the people who have joined me at different stages of this journey. I have decided that the rest of my journey will be focussed on the act of giving and sharing all that I have.

## Journals

I started journaling at the age of 13. I learned to read when I was 9 and when the world of literature opened to me, I enjoyed reading about people who went on journeys of learning. I remember reading "I am David" by Ann Holm, and feeling so many emotions about the mother who he searched for. I was inspired to self-reflect and had always wanted to be useful.

As I described earlier, I had suffered much racism as a child. I prayed in our primary school assembly, that Allah take me away from cruel people. That night, I dreamed of a beautiful white building with a flat roof and a high wall. I decided then, that Allah had a purpose for me. I began journaling my thoughts and ideas. I kept them in a nook behind my bed. I wrote about all my events and journeys. I liked to journal with pictures, then. I continued to trust that I would find that white building one day. I saw that dream again a few times but kept searching for the white building. I never found that building, only similar ones. 20 years later I got married. It was an arranged marriage. I never spoke to my fiancé. I trusted Allah from a dream about him and agreed to marry him. When I got married, I left all my journals at home. Soon after marriage, my husband suggested that we visit his family in Pakistan. When we arrived in his town, the taxi parked across the road from his house. My eyes welled with tears, as I saw the white building of my dreams. I thought about how I had journaled all my thoughts and trusted that one day they would make sense and I would find my heaven in that place of my dreams. I realise now how perfectly he was the answer to my dream since through him, I have learned to face my true self and understand my true personality rather than the fictional character I wanted to be.

In my journals, I wrote reflections of what occurred each day. I wrote about my friends and relatives. I wrote about my positive and negative experiences. I hoped that one day Allah would have mercy on me and take me to that beautiful place. I wanted to be ready. I wanted to be the best of who I was. My Dyslexia, my glasses, my teeth and then brace, my colour, my ethnicity and mixed culture, and my name were all part of my strange identity. I had felt like a misfit everywhere.

Many counsellors encourage journaling in different ways. It is a very powerful way to self-reflect. You can read what you have written and reflect on it. You will learn from what you write much more than you will from reading what I have written.

## Articles

By writing articles, I was forced to edit what I had written. By editing, I learned what were my useful, creative thoughts and what were my destructive thoughts. I realised that useful articles needed to be positive. The reader deserves the opportunity to grow by reading your article. I wrote for community magazines and was entrusted in editorial positions. I read articles written by some other authors and enabled them to write powerful, positive articles.

## Poetry

Society does not value poetry the way it was. At the time of the advent of Islam, the Arabs were famous for their poetry. The Holy Quran was described by the Meccans as a collection of poetry. There have been many great poets in history. When poetry was put to music, the attraction of music created songs and ballads.

As a child I enjoyed singing and, being in the choir, I was singing very meaningful songs and hymns and ballads. I also sang Islamic poems and was trained to sing well. Singing is very therapeutic. Unfortunately, modern, popular music is focussed mostly on party, dance music. Often, young people do not know the lyrics and when they realise the lyrics, they no longer like to listen to some of the songs because of some vulgarities or social injustices included in the lyrics. I still write poems and promote poetry writing when I teach. My children are more reflective and may read poems and enjoy the deep thoughts, emotions and imagery.

## Discussions

Every faith community promotes discussion groups and some hold inter-faith discussions. When I discuss various issues with people, almost always, the discussion revolves around love, trust, fear and grief. When you talk in a focussed group, you are able to organise your thoughts and filter what you want to share and what is private or embarrassing. One-on-one discussions can tempt you to share more than you want to and can result in regrettable conversations. Often, therapy can be a negative activity because you regret how much you have revealed about yourself. Group therapy is more productive for the simple reason that you are very actively editing your thoughts before you speak. I feel that the process is more in my control and I learn more from the experience. Individual discussions with a close friend or relative or your life partner are very important because when you reveal the truth, you can make progress in your life and the relationship. The most powerful conversations I have are when I speak to Allah in the prostration part of my daily prayers. We learn how to have these conversations when we talk to our parents as infants. We learn to trust their guidance and opinions. We learn that parents want the best for us. When we are children, we learn to pray and have those conversations with Allah. If we focus well, we see Allah's response. My children have always shared with me the responses they have witnessed from Allah in their dreams or in events in their daily lives.

## MY PRAYER FOR YOU

I hope and trust that you are now ready to embark on your *jihad*. Focus on what it is that is disturbing you and taking you off the path of righteousness. I trust that I have shared enough knowledge with you to arm you with the knowledge necessary to win your battle against fear and grief. This is my intention for this book.

At this point, my friends, I pray that Allah guide you clearly and keep you on the path of the righteous and away from those who oppose or displease the Most Loving, Forgiving, Allah.

## THE GREATER JIHAD

*"Salvation means that a person should
commit himself wholly to God,
and should offer himself as a sacrifice in the cause of God,
and should prove his sincerity not only through his motive but
also through righteous conduct.
He who so comports himself will have his recompense from God.*
 **Such people shall have no fear nor shall they grieve"** *(2:113).*

# REFLECTING ON HOW TO MANAGE FEAR AND GRIEF

# THE ABILITY TO REFLECT AND SELF-REFORM

We have recognised that there are several different aspects of our lifestyle which need to be adapted for a change in our lives. We have recognised that this is a life-long process. There is no quick fix. Our life-mission is to become faithful and hence we will not fear or grieve beyond what is necessary for our humanity.

If you are in a situation whereby you are overwhelmed and require a change for your physical and mental well-being, then this is the time to devise a plan. Allah describes that our weakest state is the state in which we may be tempted to do wrong. Allah narrates in the Holy Quran that the Prophet Joseph (peace be upon him) said to Pharaoh; CH 12 verse54

*'And I do not hold my own self to be free from weakness; for, the soul is surely prone to enjoin evil, save that whereon my Lord has mercy. Surely, my Lord is Most Forgiving, Merciful.'*

The plan for successful freedom from fear and grief requires a reflecting soul able to self-reform. Allah reminds us in the Holy Quran (CH 75 verse 3).

*And I do call to witness the self-accusing soul, that the Day of Judgment is a certainty.*

As a faithful person, you are able to reproach yourself and consider a plan which requires reflection and understanding. I will, humbly suggest some steps which you can apply to your plan. I will also suggest some journaling ideas and charts which will enable you to monitor your growth. I am not an expert in psychology, but I have seen many students and colleagues and friends and family benefit from this practical approach. I am happy to share my ideas if it will benefit you.

## 1.Pray

Since this plan is for the purpose of self-reform, which is exactly what Allah wants from us, it is logical that we ask Allah for help. Firstly, we need to consider what is the nature of our reform. If we want to become more loving, we will beg to *Al-Wadood* (The Loving Allah) If we need to repent, we will beg to *Al-Ghaffoor* (the Forgiving Allah) and so there are 100 attributes and we must tune into the wavelength of the appropriate attributes of Allah. Begging Allah by His appropriate attribute enables us to do that. This way all our actions will have the power of Allah behind us. In our prayer, we must beg to the Lord of all the worlds and beg Him to forgive us for our previous misunderstandings and ignorance as well as our mistakes. We must declare our plan for reform and beg Him for help in our planning and execution of our plan for reform. As a Muslim, we can pray for this in the state of prostration. As a Muslim, we have washed ourselves by the steps of ablution and stated our intentions before we pray. We have prayed the prescribed prayer and are able to focus completely on harnessing the love and power of Allah for our purpose.

## 2.Set Goals

Our next step is to set realistic goals with a realistic time-frame. This is what a teacher would call a long-range plan. For this, we can use a diary, or calendar or a chart such as the one below. In the diary, we can consider health and fitness, intellectual life, emotional life, character, spiritual life, relationships, social life, and financial life. If each aspect is engaged in the goal, then this holistic approach can achieve lasting results, as I myself have witnessed. These categories support the assertion of Abraham Maslow that for maximum effectiveness a person must address a hierarchy of needs.

**Fig 2.0 Maslow's Hierarchy of Needs.**

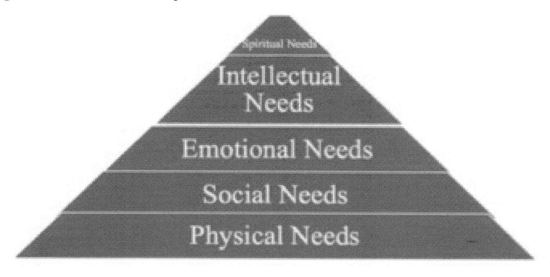

This pyramid of needs was founded on physical needs, then emotional needs, social needs, intellectual needs and then at the peak the spiritual needs. It has also been suggested that this pyramid should be reversed since it is the spirit which drives us to live.

It really is your choice what you include in your list depending on your goals and priorities. The key is that they must be doable goals within a manageable time-frame.

Determine the number of weeks by the number of steps needed to achieve the goal. You can even grade yourself so that you are actively reflecting on your achievements and how well you sustain them. By reviewing the chart, you can remind yourself of how well you did and can move on with confidence. This is what I did when I was thirteen. I continued this personal assessment and *jihad* until I was 27.

**Fig 2.1 Planning**

| Week | Emotion or Feeling | Goal | Action | Scriptural Reading/ Prayer |
|------|--------------------|------|--------|----------------------------|
| 1 Nov - 7Nov | Regret, Shame | Mend a friendship | Plan how I will meet my friend to start talking. | Prayer for forgiveness. |
| 7Nov- 14Nov | Shame | Mend a friendship | Contact my friend. | Prayer for forgiveness. |

## 3.Strategies to Stay Focussed

### Meditation

Prayer is natural to a believer, but the depth of involvement in prayer may depend on the stresses on them. As I described earlier, Allah knows how we are easily distracted. To increase our level of enjoyment of prayer, we can practice meditation. Perhaps add Yoga to the meditation time. I never appreciated the practice of Yoga until I started to practice it. Holding each pose for a few seconds while concentrating on breathing challenges the body and channels our energy. It is an excellent way to relax but more importantly, Yoga enables the mind to focus on personal needs and redirects energy. Some therapists combine Yoga with CBT. By meditating, we are able to prepare our mind for change.

### Stay Physically Fit

As I have discussed earlier, what we eat and drink and how we physically engage our body can significantly affect our ability to cope with mental health issues. This can also be planned carefully. In my family, we plan the menu for the week and then make the grocery list so that we have all the ingredients. The grocery trip is highly organized and very quick. I ensure that the grocery trip is at a time in the week when few people are shopping, so that, usually, no time is wasted in line-ups, which is stressful.

**Fig 2.2 Meal Plan**

| Day and Date | Lunch (Including School/ Work Lunch) | Dinner |
|---|---|---|
| Monday 1st | Egg sandwich/salad | Zucchini curry and rice |
| Tuesday 2nd | Veggie pasta | Chicken roast and salad |

The menu carefully includes all the food groups and balances lunch and dinner, while considering constraints such as specific dietary needs, facility to warm-up the meal at school or work and how it will be carried around and, of course consider that some foods may trigger allergic reactions in people who we sit with at a meal time.

Our other scheduled family event is the use of our family gym in our garage. Previously, we would schedule trips to our gym. At the gym, we had charts to help us regulate the fitness workout routine. I count the number of squats or crunches and other exercises which I choose for my routine. This is specific to the type of training which I am engaged in. I record the weights that I use to see how I progress and increase my fitness and stamina.

A few weeks ago, I was not able to rotate my arms for more than 4 repetitions but now I can do 15. This makes me feel really accomplished in the morning and launches a happy day. I like to keep my record cards so that I can feel good about myself and that certainly releases some serotonin in my body as well as endorphins from the exercise, which is our aim in this *jihad*.

## Restructure Our Social Network

As I presented earlier, it is very important to consider who we interact with. Some relationships are obviously toxic and need a lot of work to detoxify. You are not ready for that until you are in full control of your own emotions. Some relationships are suffering because the friend or relative is themselves in an emotional crisis and is usually indulging in negative thoughts. Some friendships or relatives are a waste of time because you are just an accessory or another name on their huge contact list. We gain little or nothing but distraction from life because of them. Social media has made this a modern disease.

Our social network needs to be positive and creative. Our friends and relatives may be many in number, but the active relationships should all be positive and creative for our recovery and reform. It is important to consider how we choose our friends or social network:

## Fig 2.4 Choosing a Suitable Companion.

| My Favorable Qualities | My Unfavorable Traits | What Qualities Can I Benefit from in a Friend? |
|---|---|---|
| I am chatty | I am a poor listener | Patience and tolerance |
| I am caring | I can be controlling | Compassionate |
| I love food | I don't like cooking | A good cook or someone who can teach me. |

# 4.Strategies To Start A Growth Spurt

## Clean-Up Our Memory Bank

Our actions may be very distant to our intentions. The most creative state is when are actions are coherent with our intentions since we are being completely sincere. For this process we must be able to forgive and move on. We do not need to tell the person that we forgive them or engage in any action. This act of forgiving is for our own peace of mind.

## Fig 2.5 Forgive

| Who or what needs to be forgiven? | What specific act needs to be forgiven? | How do I feel about the event? What are the emotions? | What will I gain by forgiving? |
|---|---|---|---|
| A boy in my grade 2 class pulled my hair | Pulling my hair | Angry. Embarrassed. Belittled. Physical pain. | Strength to face aggression. |
| He called me a "Paki" | He was racist | Lonely. Frightened. Frustrated. | Understanding and compassion for others who have suffered racism |

The example I have given is an actual event that occurred with me in England in primary school. I did forgive this incident and I became more resilient as a result. Within my memory, this is my first experience of forgiveness which I consciously learned from.

## Identify Positive Emotions

 In the whole process of planning, knowing the objective is very important. It is the light at the end of the tunnel. The objective is to have a positive, growth mindset. It is useful to identify which positive emotions are desired. You can use a chart as a reference.

**Fig 2.6. Identify Emotions**

| Emotion | Benefit of the Emotion |
|---|---|
| Compassion | I can relate to others feelings |
| Love | I will feel important |

## Select a Journaling Style

When I was 13 years old, I wrote a letter to myself every New Year's Eve and assessed myself regarding some important goals. This was a very brief chart. As I grew older, I realised the need for a diary or journal where I could write about events and how I dealt with them. In the previous chapter, I have suggested various ways in which one can write. The style depends on your age, ability and opportunity to write and your learning style.

In this book, I have discussed fear and grief separately but have recognised that there are common issues as well. The next two chapters separate the two again so that you can focus on what issues are related to fear and what issues are related to grief. This is your book, so perhaps you will want to use ideas from both sections since fear can lead to grief and grief can lead to fear.

# MANAGING FEARS

## 1.Identify Exactly What Are The Fears

By identifying the emotions which you are feeling, you can engage in feeling it properly. Face the emotion. Pray or meditate about it. Journal the event and story linked with it. Avoid fighting the emotion or suppressing it. Relate to the emotions which may have been felt by the other person involved so that you can empathise. Understand how the emotion is negatively affecting you and others involved. The emotions lead to fears. If the emotions can be addressed, then the fears can be identified and noted.

## 2.Identify Which Emotions Are Engaged

At this point, it is important to identify which emotions you wish to experience so that you can grow. The emotions which you are familiar with will be in your control and enable you to grow. The emotions that you are not familiar with are new because the situation you may be facing is also new to you.

a) **Anger** implies that someone has violated your rights or that your needs have been denied or that your boundaries have been crossed.
b) **Anxiety** implies that you do not have enough information about a situation and there are some aspects which are frightening for you.

c) **Fear and Pain** implies that an event frightened you such that you fear the past. Pain is the result of you being physically violated.

d) **Sadness** implies that something precious has been lost

## 3.Identify Which Attributes of Allah are Needed

There are 100 attributes of Allah. There is certainly an attribute for any human problem. If we focus on that attribute such as the Healer (*As Shaafi*) when we embark on an activity or prayer before that activity, then we connect with Allah and find Him and His help specifically for the problem. When siblings argue, it is very painful for parents. I like to pray to Allah *Al Wadood* and pray for the siblings to find the love in their hearts to discuss the issue without hurting each other. In the Holy Quran, a hundred attributes of Allah are mentioned and described. You can select which ones are best suited to your prayer needs from the chart below. I have listed the attributes which I consider are suitable.

**Fig 2.7 Attributes of Allah**

| Attribute of Allah | Meaning |
|---|---|
| Rabbil Al Ameen | Lord of All the Worlds |
| Rehman | Gracious |
| Raheem | Merciful |
| Al Qayoom | The Self-Subsisting and All Sustaining |
| Al Wadood | The Loving |
| Al Ghuffaar | The Forgiving |
| As Sami | The All Hearing |
| Ash Shaafi | The Healer |
| As Salam | The source of Peace |
| Al Muhaimim | The Protector |
| Al Azeez | The Mighty |
| Al Khaaliq | The Creator |
| Al Aleem | The All Knowing |
| Al Baseer | The All- Seeing |
| Al Adl | The Just |
| Al Hafeez | The Guardian |
| Al Mujeeb | The Answerer (of prayers) |
| Al Hakeem | The Wise |
| Al Qadir | The Processor of Power and Authority |
| Ar Ra'oof | The Compassionate |

## 4.Set a Time-Scale

You are now ready to plan your *jihad*. There may be a deadline already set or you can set a deadline by which you can achieve the desired level of fearlessness. You have identified exactly what it is that you are fearful of. You have decided who will be supporting you through this *jihad*. You have decided what your specific goals are

**Fig 2.8 My Action Plan**

| Date | Action | Result |
|------|--------|--------|
| 3rd Nov | Check text messages from my co-worker | Found last text. She rudely asked for my work. |
| 4th Nov | Identify what she wanted to say to me. | Plan a positive and assertive response. Forgive her rude text. |

Now you can fill out this guide for your action plan. Be in full control of this mission. Pray to Allah for support in your mission.

# 5. Some Powerful Prayers and Journaling Ideas

I remember as a child that prayer books were very popular and many diaries had prayers to start each journal page. There are believers, like us who still enjoy these prayers and words of wisdom. I like to write prayers from the Holy Quran and words of wisdom or poetry in my journals. Here are some examples of prayers from the Holy Quran:

> *"Our Lord, do not punish us, if we forget or fall into error; and our Lord, lay not on us a responsibility as You did lay upon those before us; Our Lord, burden us not with what we have not the strength to bear; and efface our sins, and grant us forgiveness and have mercy on us; You are our Master; so help us You against the disbelieving people."* CH2 Verse 287

> *Our Lord, in You do we put our trust, and to You do we turn repentant, and towards You is the final return.* Ch 60 verse 5

> *You are our Protector; forgive us then, and have mercy on us, for You are the Best of those who forgive* CH 7 verse 156

> *Lord, I have indeed wronged my soul, therefore, forgive me.* CH 28 verse 17

> *My Lord, open up for me my heart. And ease for me my task. And untie the knot of my tongue, that they may understand my speech.* CH 20 verses 26-29O

*My Lord, a beggar I am of whatever good You bestow upon me.* CH28 Verse 25

*I am overcome, so come Thou to my help.* CH 45 verse11

*My Lord, my people have treated me as a liar. Therefore, judge You decisively between them and me and save me and the believers that are with me.* CH 26 verses 118-119

*Help me, my Lord, against the wicked people.* CH29 verse 31

*My Lord, save me and my family from what they do.* CH 26 verse 170

*My Lord, bestow wisdom on me and join me with the righteous; and give me a true reputation among posterity; and make me one of the inheritors of the Garden of Bliss.* CH26 verses 84-86

*Sufficient for us is Allah, and an excellent Guardian.* Ch3 verse 174

*Surely, to Allah we belong and to Him shall we return.* CH2 verse 175

*Allah is sufficient for me. There is no God but He. In Him do I put my trust, and He is the Lord of the Mighty Throne.* CH9 verse 129

*In the name of Allah, the Gracious, the Merciful. Say, 'I seek refuge in the Lord of mankind, the King of mankind, the God of mankind, from the evil of the sneaking whisperer, who whispers into the hearts of men, from among the Jinn and mankind.* CH 114 verses 1-7

For all of these prayers, it is best if they are reflected upon and said with conviction that Allah is listening. Ablution performed in the same way as before the daily prayers enhances the effectiveness of these prayers. I like to pray whenever I feel the need, but, I also like to search for them in The Holy Quran and understand the context of them in the story narrated in the Holy Quran.

## 6.Foods and Activities for Bravery and Strength

I discussed diet earlier and described how I changed our family diet according to our family health goals. We needed to increase the happy hormones and, for that I tried to make our diet as alkali as possible. I also minimized packaged food and spices. I now try to make meals fresh and avoid storing cooked food in the fridge or freezer. By doing this, we have become stronger and more resilient. Our immune system is also stronger. Allah has guided us to a healthy human friendly diet with mostly seasonal fruit and vegetables and meats. I have also increased my understanding of the benefits of the various herbs and spices which I use.

The internet is swamped with health websites advising what food to eat for various conditions. You know best what your personal and family needs are. I can only speak for my family. It depends on your nature and your present mental condition. It is very easy to get lost in the trails of YouTube videos and health websites. It is best to begin by identifying what your deficiencies may be. Prophet Muhammad (peace be upon him) told us that "there is a cure for every disease" and so it is our strength of faith which determines how we will find the cure.

**Fig 2.9 Foods for Bravery and Strength**

| Health condition | Symptoms | Source of information (website/ video etc.) | Food, drink or herbal remedy | Benefits |
|---|---|---|---|---|
| IBS | Acute intestinal pain | | Green juice | Anti-inflammatory. Easy to digest nutrition |

There are some well-known herbs which help put you on the right track.

**Fig 2.10 Herbs for Bravery and Strength**

| Herb | Affect | How to use it |
|---|---|---|
| Ashwaghanda | Mental Strength | 1 teaspoon Powder in smoothie |
| Chamomile | Calming | Oil in diffuser or tea |
| St John's Wort | Anti-depressant | In tea |
| Poppy seeds | Anti-depressant | Energy balls |
| Melon seeds | Brains strength | Energy balls |

There are also some well-known foods which help you develop a happy positive mindset. They are usually yellow.

**Fig 2.11 Happy Foods**

| Food | Affect | How to use it |
|---|---|---|
| Bananas | Provide Potassium and Magnesium to relax body. L-Tryptophan can convert to Serotonin | Eat. Smoothie. Fruit salad. |
| Sweet potato | Anti-oxidant for the brain and the carbohydrates can help make serotonin | Fries. Mash. |

# 7.Planning The *Jihad*

The plan is to become fearless of worldly situations and fearful for our status in the after-life and the legacy we leave when we go. Since we believe that there is an after-life which we are here to prepare for, our focus is diverted to a more serious predicament. If at our last breath, we are unfulfilled and feel that we need to do many things to achieve the status we hope for in heaven, then we need to solve our worldly problems with a new energy. We need to harness that energy from the world around us. Our plan can now be fashioned around these goals.

Since you are probably reading this book; and certainly this part of the book because you need some guidance about how to liberate yourself from anxiety of fear and grief, it is essential for me to provide a template for you to base your planning ideas. This is the teacher part of my practice. I have used this method of planning as a professional teacher and also at home with my family. They may not have realised it, but my brain enjoys planning every 6 weeks. This is a comfortable time-frame to work with.

## The Long-Range Plan For 6 Weeks

This long-range plan must clearly state the learning objectives and the criteria by which you will recognise that you are making progress. Any teachers reading this are probably rolling their eyes. I believe that what we teach in school is a foundation for life skills. Otherwise it is pointless. So, let us continue and ignore the eye-rollers.

### Fig 2.13 The 6-Week Plan

| Week | Date | Objective | Success criteria |
|------|------|-----------|------------------|
| 1 | Nov 1 | Be able to walk in the park when there are dogs present. | Manage nerves when a dog walks past with its owner. |
| 2 | Nov 8 | Same | Walk at normal pace when a dog walks past with its owner. |
| 3 | Nov 15 | Same | Walk at a normal pace while looking calmly at a dog when it walks past with its owner. |

To manage anxiety related to the specific fears you may have, I would advise that you try to identify little steps by which you can overcome the fears. To identify the most important fear, make a list or brainstorm all the fears related to one event. Circle the most frightening one which cause your hands to become clammy or your heart to race, or your body to shiver or some other worrying reaction. For this event, identify the component parts of the event and list them in order. The first should be the aspect which worries you the most. In this way, you are able to address the physical needs that you have in that situation. Gradually, address aspects relating to your emotional needs, social needs, your knowledge about the event and finally how your spirit feels at that event. If each aspect is awarded adequate time and attention, then you should gradually be able to move toward an acceptance of the event and face the fears so that you gain courage and manage the event. I cannot dictate the time-span required.

You can adjust it as you progress. If you supplement the process with good nutrition, exercise, good company, prayers and reflective journaling, I believe that this is possible for anyone. This is the formula which I have applied and it works for many who believe. God willing it will work for you.

# MANAGING GRIEF

## 1.Identify Exactly What Have Been The Losses

At a time of loss, it feels as if you are the only one who feels that way and that it cannot happen to anyone else the way it happened to you. For a Muslim, Allah advises us to remember[3]

*Who, when a misfortune overtakes them, say, 'Surely, to Allah we belong and to Him shall we return.'* CH2 Vs157

This statement, in itself has such a calming effect. It reminds us that one day we will be missed and that is Devine Decree. Only Allah is permanent. However, we need strategies to cope at that immediate time of loss. Many people like to write an obituary when a loved one dies. This reminds them of how they connected with you. You can do the same for any loss and feel the same emotions when you identify exactly what you have lost. For a person who has lost their grandmother, she may have been a mother, a friend, an adviser, a mentor, a support all tied in a grandmother who has passed away.

## Fig 3.1 Losses

| What did I Lose OR<br><br>Who did I lose? | Why was it special for me?<br><br>Why were they special to me? |
|---|---|
| My ring | It was given to me by my great aunt |
| My great uncle | He was my substitute grandfather |
| My full-time job | I felt important at work and I felt strong |

## 2. Identify The Emotions And Symptoms

For each aspect of the loss, there will be different emotions. I was devastated when my father passed away. I remember laughing with family when we remembered how my father drove his car. He took us all over Europe in his cars, but he never quite understood the purpose of the clutch in the manual car. Those who drove cars before the advent of automatic transmission will know what that means. There were feelings of anger because he did not trust his doctors during the chemotherapy. There were feelings of love when we remembered how much he loved everyone and even his plants. When I journaled these feelings in my diary, it gave me immediate relief but it also gave me relief later when I re-read the journal.

## Fig 3.2 Emotions

| What Was the Loss? | How Do I Feel About It? |
|---|---|
| My father passed away | I feel like I have no one to lean on and I am alone when I want to share personal concerns or achievements. He always found the good in everything I did and believed I could do more. |

## 3.Set a Time-Scale

As with the previous chapter, it is important to allow yourself time. Although in Islam, bereavement is prescribed a time period, so that, the bereaved can move on in their life and value the moments that Allah has allowed them to live. For a bereaved wife, she is required to mourn for 40 days so that it can be established if she is pregnant and will have needs. This also enables her to present a true picture of her predicament to any potential suiter for her re-marriage. These are practical considerations. However, a bereavement can last many years and revisit the heart at different events. In order to overcome a loss, it is important to set small steps of healing.

In Islam, we are encouraged to specifically visit the grave for the first 40 days and also each Eid festival after the service and if possible, on Fridays after the service. When we are at the grave, we greet the deceased "Peace be with you O dwellers of the grave" Then, we pray for the deceased.

For other losses, our grief should be as brief as possible since then it is possible to accept the next stage and realise what we have learned from the experience.

## 4.Foods to Soothe and Heal the Heart

To bear a loss, the body needs to cool down and transmit positive messages to all the organs. In scientific terms, the body will be in a need of serotonin to replenish a sense of self-worth, dopamine for the pleasure of starting a new day and a new life, and oxytocin to ease away the pain that comes with any loss. These chemicals can be attained in some foods and herbs as well as from some actions.

Barley is an excellent source of tryptophan which the body converts into serotonin. There are other grains which are also good sources of tryptophan but barley stands out. Prophet Muhammad (peace be upon him) recommended that grieved individuals should be given *Talbina*. *Talbina* is a milky pudding made like rice pudding but with barley and sweetened with honey. I like to make this in the summer for my family since that is also a time when school ends and the kids miss their friends and also the weather is very hot. I also like to take some for grieving families when I visit.

Sweet potatoes and other foods are also a good source of tryptophan. Nutritionists have identified many foods which have specific properties to calm the brain and heart and enable the mind to think in a more positive way or at least to focus on the present and enable you to deal with your daily needs so that you can build the strength to address your fears and grief. In my family there are some key diet changes which have enabled us to deal with the challenges and events of life. I will not prescribe any specific herbs or foods since I am not a nutritionist or naturopath. However, I would recommend that you certainly look at what you eat. Allah says in the Holy Quran

*'Eat of the good things that We have provided for you, and transgress not therein, lest My wrath descend upon you; and he on whom My wrath descends shall perish;* (20:82)

**Fig 3.3 Foods to Heal**

| Food/Herb/Drink | How It Is Useful | How to Use It |
|---|---|---|
| Barley | Tryptophan makes serotonin to reduce anxiety and depression. | Make a milky pudding with honey and coarse organic barley flour. |
| Ashwaghanda | Reduces depressive symptoms and gives strength | 1 teaspoon of organic powder in a smoothie |

I like to begin the day with a juice a ginger juice. I juice one apple with a 1-inch piece of ginger. This is a great formula of how to deal with negative emotions. First, eliminate the toxins and then build strength.

### 5. Activities To Soothe And Heal The Heart

The first activity for grief is to recite the prayer

*'Surely, to Allah we belong and to Him shall we return.'[4]*

I often advise my family members that even if they have lost a pencil, they can recite this prayer and be at peace with the loss. This will increase resilience. I have seen mothers struggle with children in toy stores, when they cannot cope with leaving without a new toy. This is usually because the child feels that the purchase assures them that their mother loves them and the protest is not as much for the toy as it is for the reassurance that they have not lost the love of their mother. I was aware of this when my children were very young. The prayer also promotes gratitude for the life, people and things that they have.

Meet others and talk about the loss with a friend or relative. This activity ensures that you do not feel that you are alone and that nobody else would understand how you feel. For bereavement, Islam prescribes that for the first few days friends and neighbors visit and express their sympathies and listen and pray and recite the Holy Quran together. Community members can help to console the bereaved family. For other losses also, it is helpful to share your experience and grief. You will be able to express your emotions and calm down. Some people feel embarrassed about their emotions as if it is only children and weak women who are permitted to cry. All humans have tear glands and a soul. When the soul is aggrieved, it should be allowed to express emotions. That is better relief for the heart.

This is a time to be with a group of loved ones who you can trust and confide in. whatever your loss is, it is not enough to just pray. Allah has made us live in communities so that we learn to love and care and be compassionate and grateful and so many more positive emotions and feelings which develop our growth mindset.

*And We bestowed wisdom on Luqman, saying, 'Be grateful to Allah:' and whoso is grateful, is grateful only for the good of his own soul. And whoso is ungrateful, then surely Allah is Self-Sufficient, Praiseworthy.*
CH31 Verse 13

In my community, the members are organised so that each country is divided into regions and towns and chapters. Each chapter has up to 200 members who are managed by a leader who cares for all the needs of members regularly with a team of volunteers. It is almost impossible for any member to be ignored and there is always someone who can help.

In most communities, there are help groups who are often voluntary or not-for-profit. These organisations are driven by a strong sense of compassion which brings them together. If one cannot help you, they will know of another who can. There is so much love to be found that there is no reason to suffer alone.

It is your choice which group you choose to contact. The activity can only be a positive one. However sometimes the loss is due to a negative behaviour which makes you unapproachable since you may have lost your temper or behaved in an aggressive manner.

**The 4 Step Problem Solving Strategy**.

As a teacher, I like to work with students on strategies which will enable them to overcome difficulties when I am not there to help them. The four steps needed to solve social problems which lead to loss of social acceptance and grief are very simple to follow.

   **I. Define the problem.** Be completely honest about what exactly the problem is.

   **II. Create and consider a solution.** Consider how to solve the immediate problem yourself. It is very easy to say what others can do. You cannot make someone do something. You can only make yourself do something or model it for someone else through your own actions.

**III. Implement a solution.** When you have a plan, execute it as soon as possible. You may modify it as you implement it but persevere with Allah's help.

**IV. Make an agreement.** By taking some action, you have shown the most important emotion. You have expressed that you are disappointed that it happened and that you want to correct it so that you do not lose the relationship jeopardised by the incident.

**Fig 3.4 Problem-Solving**

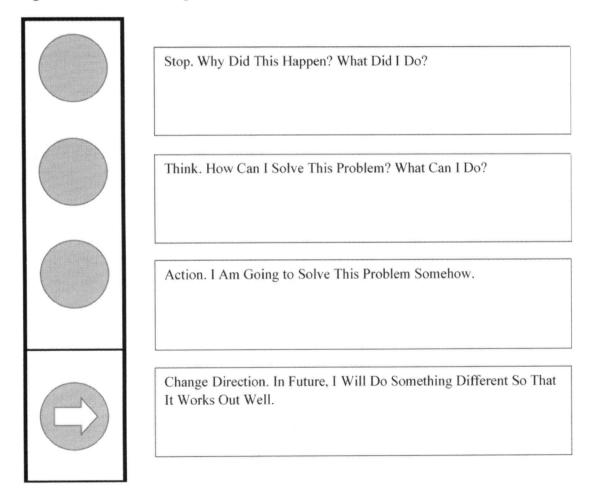

Stop. Why Did This Happen? What Did I Do?

Think. How Can I Solve This Problem? What Can I Do?

Action. I Am Going to Solve This Problem Somehow.

Change Direction. In Future, I Will Do Something Different So That It Works Out Well.

| Stop | It is upsetting when family do not join for dinner when I call them repeatedly |
|---|---|
| Think | I can set dinner time at 7:30pm or a time when everyone is home and ready. |
| Action | I talk to the whole family about my plan and why it is important to me. |
| Change | We agree as a family on family meal times and chores so all are involved. |

Often, terrible situations can be avoided by adjusting the way we think. The way we think may be a very old bad habit which will require a process to change. This process requires us to recognise the errors in our way of thinking.

## Adjusting Our Thinking

### Exaggerating

Sometimes, we can exaggerate the intensity of an issue. Moms yell at children when they spill something and ignore the fact that the child spilled water which can easily be cleaned up. In the process, mom has missed the fact that her child was trying to be independent and this may have been a landmark in his learning. Mom has lost the flowers in the vase but must really grieve more at the loss of a learning opportunity.

### Negative View

Our view may habitually be negative. As above, mom could have laughed with the child about the flowers, rescued them and appreciated the child for caring to add water for the care of the flowers.

### Black and White

A compassionate heart sees the world as many colours where a goal can be achieved in many ways. A compassionate heart is forgiving. A compassionate heart can see new opportunities. To move away from black and white thinking, the heart must try to become compassionate. It is a very rewarding and healthy change.

**Pessimist.**

It is productive to deal with each unique event and solve each problem as it comes. Wisdom, may indicate that there is a trend but should not dictate what will occur in the future. If grandma and mother died of breast cancer, statistics will dictate that that is your future, but the growth mindset decides that they will change the statistics. I have seen that happen myself. It is Allah's will.

**Personalising.**

It is very easy to feel that you are to blame in a negative and often counter-productive way. Millions of people are facing loss at the same time every day. Various circumstances lead to those losses and insurance companies make a lot of money out of it. It is healthier to consider what you can learn from the event and find out how other people learn from it. Laying the blame on anyone is counter-productive. Laying the blame on yourself is only affective if you plan to do something to reform yourself.

**Blame Others.**

It is also very easy to blame others for your mistakes. You can only change yourself. It is pointless to blame others who you cannot change.

## 6. Tracking the Healing Process

As with the previous chapter, I would recommend that you track your own process of healing from a loss. You can add detail or ideas of your own to suit your style of journaling. The objective is to solve problems of grieving which are affecting your health and your ability to function in your daily life. Grief can be very isolating and demoralising. This is a personal *jihad* which will strengthen your heart and resilience.

Through this journey, you will learn how all things are temporary and so it is healthier to enjoy things while you have them and objectively address the loss after they go. If this idea is instilled in children, then live is a smoother ride. In my childhood, death was a taboo for children and so we never attended funerals or burials. I know of one dear friend who has daughters who are involved in the preparation of the deceased for burial and have been doing this since they were 16 years old. When you are able to detach yourself from worldly needs and desires, your level of gratitude and acceptance will increase and every event will be appreciated in a positive way. This is the objective and success will lead to resilience

## Fig 3.5 Tracking the Healing Process

| Week | Date | Objective | Success Criteria |
|---|---|---|---|
| 1 | Nov 1 | Cope with leaving of my job | Finish all matters related to my job. Bring home personal items. Clean work area. |
| 2 | Nov 8 | Understand why I was fired | Be able to articulate what lead to the event. |
| 3 | Nov 15 | Cope with leaving old friends | Speak to all friends and arrange how you will keep in touch. Find items which remind you of them. |

# PLANNING THE 6 STEPS

## 1. The Goal of this Journey

The goal of this journey is peace of mind. As I suggested earlier, peace of mind is achieved when you detach yourself from worldly matters. I like to focus on two main aspects of my life. One is the mark I make on the world I leave behind. The other is the life I desire after my death which has been promised to us by Allah. Fear and grief are mostly rooted in the world. We learn these two negative emotions from our worldly experiences. Allah has given many examples throughout history in all cultures of how people who were too attached to the world became fearful and made huge losses. Some repented at their last breath. What a waste of a life!

I have tried to share a 6-step formula which has been successful so far in my life. I was so delighted at the results that I felt the need to share it with you. Some of it may seem naïve or obvious. I do believe that we have a lot to learn from the obvious and naïve. I enjoy teaching children because actually they teach me more than I teach them. We learn together how to build a better future. The future I desire for the world is one where we are all able to live together with compassion and love. I desire that we leave judgement to Allah and think well of each other. I believe that the world needs to learn to forgive the past, appreciate the variety of gifts we all have to offer and share those gifts as a way of gratitude and worship to Allah.

There will be critics who may ask how I am qualified to write this book. They will say that there could be more content and knowledge. I wanted to share my experience of how Islam is the solution to problems. I wanted to start my reader thinking with a growth mindset knowing that there is a manual to help you. That manual may be the Holy Quran, but may be any other scripture that was from our Creator.

May Allah Bless you all in your quest for a positive mindset.

# JOURNAL

Pages from this journal may be copied to create your own personal journal pages. More ideas are available on my website.

## Journal

This journal is intended to enable you to embark on a journey of self-reflection guided by our Creator. It is your personal journey. Be completely sincere and frank with yourself.

Through self-reflection, prayer, consultation with loved ones and journaling, you will realise your true purpose, strengths and realistic ambitions. You will now be able to self-reform your thinking, actions and beliefs about yourself and your relationships. May Allah be your guide. Ameen.

*"Salvation means that a person should*

*commit himself wholly to God,*

*and should offer himself as a sacrifice in the cause of God,*

*and should prove his sincerity not only through his motive but also through righteous conduct.*

*He who so comports himself will have his recompense from God.*

***Such people shall have no fear nor shall they grieve"*** *(2:113).*

# My Fears or Grief

List the most problematic fears or griefs or both. How do they each affect your daily function?

| What Is My Fear or Grief? | How Is It Affecting Me? |
|---|---|
| | |
| | |
| | |
| | |
| | |

## What Are My Most Important Concerns?

| What I Am Most Concerned About | How Is It Impacting My Health? | How Is It Impacting My Relationships? | How Is It Impacting My Faith? |
|---|---|---|---|
|  |  |  |  |
|  |  |  |  |
|  |  |  |  |
|  |  |  |  |
|  |  |  |  |
|  |  |  |  |

## Strength of Faith and Spirit

Setting time for prayer or meditation is challenging when there are other duties and needs. A Muslim is required to pray 5 times a day.

| Date | Dawn | Mid-day | Afternoon | Dusk | Night |
|------|------|---------|-----------|------|-------|
|      |      |         |           |      |       |
|      |      |         |           |      |       |
|      |      |         |           |      |       |
|      |      |         |           |      |       |
|      |      |         |           |      |       |
|      |      |         |           |      |       |
|      |      |         |           |      |       |
|      |      |         |           |      |       |
|      |      |         |           |      |       |
|      |      |         |           |      |       |
|      |      |         |           |      |       |
|      |      |         |           |      |       |
|      |      |         |           |      |       |

| Attribute of Allah | Meaning |
| --- | --- |
| Rabbil Al Ameen | Lord of All the Worlds |
| Rehman | Gracious |
| Raheem | Merciful |
| Al Qayoom | The Self-Subsisting and All Sustaining |
| Al Wadood | The Loving |
| Al Ghuffaar | The Forgiving |
| As Sami | The All Hearing |
| Ash Shaafi | The Healer |
| As Salam | The source of Peace |
| Al Muhaimim | The Protector |
| Al Azeez | The Mighty |
| Al Khaaliq | The Creator |
| Al Aleem | The All Knowing |
| Al Baseer | The All- Seeing |
| Al Adl | The Just |
| Al Hafeez | The Guardian |
| Al Mujeeb | The Answerer (of prayers) |
| Al Hakeem | The Wise |
| Al Qadir | The Processor of Power and Authority |
| Ar Ra'oof | The Compassionate |
| | |
| | |
| | |
| | |

# Reading Scripture

Reading scripture is a great launch to the day.

| Date | Scripture | What I Read About | What I Learned | How I Can Apply This Today |
|------|-----------|-------------------|----------------|----------------------------|
|      |           |                   |                |                            |
|      |           |                   |                |                            |
|      |           |                   |                |                            |
|      |           |                   |                |                            |
|      |           |                   |                |                            |
|      |           |                   |                |                            |
|      |           |                   |                |                            |

## My Physical Health and Strength

I have discussed the importance of physical strength and health. Over a few weeks, you can monitor how you get stronger by improving the aspects listed.

| Date | My Weight | My Hours of Sleep | My Hours of Leisure or Rest | My Hours of Physical Activity | My Hours of Time with Significant Relationships | How Many Litres of Water I Drank |
|------|-----------|-------------------|------------------------------|-------------------------------|--------------------------------------------------|----------------------------------|
|      |           |                   |                              |                               |                                                  |                                  |
|      |           |                   |                              |                               |                                                  |                                  |
|      |           |                   |                              |                               |                                                  |                                  |
|      |           |                   |                              |                               |                                                  |                                  |
|      |           |                   |                              |                               |                                                  |                                  |
|      |           |                   |                              |                               |                                                  |                                  |
|      |           |                   |                              |                               |                                                  |                                  |
|      |           |                   |                              |                               |                                                  |                                  |
|      |           |                   |                              |                               |                                                  |                                  |
|      |           |                   |                              |                               |                                                  |                                  |
|      |           |                   |                              |                               |                                                  |                                  |
|      |           |                   |                              |                               |                                                  |                                  |
|      |           |                   |                              |                               |                                                  |                                  |
|      |           |                   |                              |                               |                                                  |                                  |

# Foods and Supplements which will Support my Mental Health

Everyone is different and have specific needs and reactions to these foods and herbs.It is our duty to find it and then to use it properly with conviction. Often people buy the remedies but only use it for a few days and then give up. Please persevere, and if one is not effective, then try another.

| My Health Condition | My Symptoms | Source of Information (Nutritionist, Naturopath, Website/ Video Etc.) | Food, Drink or Herbal Remedy | Benefits for Me |
|---|---|---|---|---|
|  |  |  |  |  |
|  |  |  |  |  |
|  |  |  |  |  |
|  |  |  |  |  |
|  |  |  |  |  |
|  |  |  |  |  |

## My Diet Plan

Plan a balanced menu for the week to include all the essential foods to support your mental health.

| Day and Date | Lunch | Dinner |
|---|---|---|
|  |  |  |
|  |  |  |
|  |  |  |
|  |  |  |
|  |  |  |
|  |  |  |
|  |  |  |

# Cleanliness and Massage

Before each prayer, a Muslim believer washes by a set routine. This includes light massage of each part of the body. To begin this habit, concentrate on one part for each prayer or meditation time. Note which part of the body enjoyed a massage.

| Date | Dawn | Mid-Day | Afternoon | Dusk | Night |
|------|------|---------|-----------|------|-------|
|  |  |  |  |  |  |
|  |  |  |  |  |  |
|  |  |  |  |  |  |
|  |  |  |  |  |  |
|  |  |  |  |  |  |
|  |  |  |  |  |  |
|  |  |  |  |  |  |
|  |  |  |  |  |  |
|  |  |  |  |  |  |
|  |  |  |  |  |  |
|  |  |  |  |  |  |
|  |  |  |  |  |  |

# Exercise

| Body/machine | Setting/pose | weight | reps | Time | date |
|---|---|---|---|---|---|
| Warm up | | | | | |
| Head and shoulders | | | | | |
| | | | | | |
| | | | | | |
| | | | | | |
| | | | | | |
| Cardio | | | | | |
| Cool down | | | | | |

# My Social and Emotional Strength

| My Favorable Qualities | My Unfavorable Traits | What Qualities Can I Benefit from In A Friend. |
|---|---|---|
| | | |
| | | |
| | | |
| | | |
| | | |
| | | |
| | | |

# Positive Emotions

In the accompanying book, I have discussed some positive emotions. Try to list others as you discover them.

| Emotion | Benefit of the Emotion |
|---|---|
| Compassion | I can relate to other's feelings |
| Love | I will feel important |
|  |  |
|  |  |
|  |  |
|  |  |
|  |  |
|  |  |
|  |  |

# Negative Emotions

List the negative emotions which you want to be free of.

| Emotion | How This Emotion Has Hurt You |
|---|---|
|  |  |
|  |  |
|  |  |

# My Ability to Forgive

Event:

| Who or what needs to be forgiven? | What specific act needs to be forgiven? | How do I feel about the event? What are the emotions? | What will I gain by forgiving? |
|---|---|---|---|
| | | | |
| | | | |
| | | | |
| | | | |
| | | | |
| | | | |
| | | | |

# My losses

| What was the loss? | How do I feel about it? |
| --- | --- |
|  |  |
|  |  |
|  |  |

| What was the loss? | How do I feel about it? |
| --- | --- |
|  |  |
|  |  |
|  |  |

| What was the loss? | How do I feel about it? |
| --- | --- |
|  |  |
|  |  |
|  |  |

## My Social Action Plan

When anxious, it is very easy in that stressful state, to upset or offend someone who you care about. So many upsets can be avoided. Try this action plan to resolve the situation.

| | |
|---|---|
| Stop | |
| Think | |
| Action | |
| Change | |

| | |
|---|---|
| Stop | |
| Think | |
| Action | |
| Change | |

| | |
|---|---|
| Stop | |
| Think | |
| Action | |
| Change | |

## My Plan

Over the next 6 weeks, I want to:

| Week | Date | Objective | Success Criteria |
|---|---|---|---|
| | | | |
| | | | |
| | | | |
| | | | |
| | | | |
| | | | |

SHEILA MALIK

| | Monday | Tuesday | Wednesday | Thursday | Friday | Saturday | Sunday |
|---|---|---|---|---|---|---|---|
| 1 | | | | | | | |
| 2 | | | | | | | |
| 3 | | | | | | | |
| 4 | | | | | | | |
| 5 | | | | | | | |
| 6 | | | | | | | |

| date | My goal today | My successes | I need to work on... |
|---|---|---|---|
| | | | |
| | | | |
| | | | |
| | | | |
| | | | |
| | | | |
| | | | |

---

[1] Sabians refers to anyone who has turned to the One God.

[2] La hawla wala quwwata illa billa

[3] *"inna lillah wa inna ilayhe rajeoon"*

[4] "Inna lillah wa inna ilayhe rajeoon."

Manufactured by Amazon.ca
Bolton, ON

32436564R00063